CANDIDA
ALBICANS

By the same author:

The Acupuncture Treatment of Pain
Amino Acids in Therapy
Soft-Tissue Manipulation

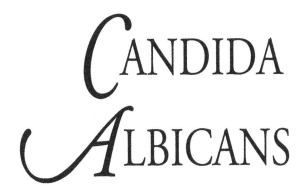

CANDIDA ALBICANS

Could

Yeast

Be Your

Problem?

LEON CHAITOW, D.O., N.D.

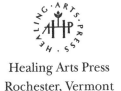

Healing Arts Press
Rochester, Vermont

Healing Arts Press
One Park Street
Rochester, Vermont 05767
www.InnerTraditions.com

This revised and expanded edition published by Healing Arts Press in 1998
Copyright © 1998 by Leon Chaitow

*Note to the reader: This book is intended as an informational guide. The remedies,
approaches, and techniques described herein are meant to supplement, and not to be a
substitute for, professional medical care or treatment. They should not be used to treat a
serious ailment without prior consultation with a qualified health-care professional.*

LIBRARY OF CONGRESS CATALOGING-IN-PUBLICATION DATA

Chaitow, Leon.
Candida albicans : could yeast be your problem? / Leon Chaitow. — Rev. and expanded ed.
p. cm.
Includes bibliographical references and index.
ISBN 978-0-89281-795-5
1. Candidiasis—Popular works. 2. Candida albicans—Popular works. I. Title.
RC123.C3C48   1998   98-18448
616.9'69—dc21   CIP

Printed and bound in the United States

10 9 8

Healing Arts Press is a division of Inner Traditions International

CONTENTS

Acknowledgements

The pioneering research of Dr C. Orion Truss in the uncovering of Candida's involvement in a wide range of diseases and conditions deserves recognition. I would respectfully dedicate this book to him. Others who have made major contributions to this knowledge, and to whom I owe a debt, include Dr William G. Crook and Dr Jeffrey Bland. I have quoted from all three of these respected scientists, and thank them on behalf of all those who will benefit from their original work. The books of Dr Truss and Dr Crook (*The Missing Diagnosis* and *The Yeast Connection*, respectively – see Further Information) are worthy of study by anyone who wishes to have a deeper knowledge of this subject.

Chapter 1
CANDIDA YEAST AND
COMMON HEALTH PROBLEMS

In the past ten years or so it has become clear that a surprising number of common health problems, both physical and mental, might have a common cause – namely, the spread in the body of a yeast that lives in each and every one of us. Its name is *Candida Albicans*, and I will call it Candida for short.

Since the first edition of this book (published in 1985) the major emphasis in my practice has involved people with Candida overgrowth and its associated health problems, such as chronic allergy and chronic fatigue (ME). The degree of the problem world-wide has become increasingly apparent to me as a result of the stream of letters which continually arrives from readers of this book. Many contain phrases such as 'this book has changed my life,' and often come with heartbreaking stories of desperate health situations which have been positively transformed (although not overnight) by the application of its principles. While receiving such letters is truly humbling, the real credit should go to the pioneers of research into the subject, such as Dr C. Orion Truss of Alabama, USA, who first noticed what no one else seemed able to see, although it was staring them in the face. Because it is present in all people from the first few months of life, Candida tends to be overlooked by doctors seeking the causes of particular diseases or conditions. Since it is present in everyone, it seems that they think that Candida could not possibly be causing the wide range of symptoms which are now linked to yeast overgrowth in so many people. This reasoning has prevented medical attention being given to Candida, except in rare conditions in which it proliferates to such an extent as to become life-threatening, something which often happens in people whose defence mechanism (immune system) has become weakened by disease or drugs (whether these are used in therapy or are abused). This may help us to understand why a great many people suffer from a less pronounced spread of Candida, which, although usually not severe enough to endanger life, is certainly sufficient to produce a wide array of often debilitating symptoms which can include:

- depression
- anxiety
- unnatural irritability
- digestive symptoms such as diarrhoea, constipation, bloating and heartburn
- extreme fatigue and a sense of hopelessness
- an inability to concentrate ('brain-fog')
- allergies
- acne
- migraine
- widespread muscular pain
- cystitis
- vaginitis
- thrush
- menstrual problems and pre-menstrual tension.

Understanding the way in which this wide range of symptoms can result from the effects of a yeast that lives in all of us, demands that we appreciate those factors which will encourage a spread of yeast in anyone. In most people there is an uneasy truce between the body and the yeasts that live inside it. Over many thousands of years a balance has been struck. Yeast can live, and thrive, and present no problems to its host, the body, as long as it confines itself to specific sites. Should it go beyond these sites, the defence capability of the body, as represented by its immune system in general and its white blood cells in particular, attacks and destroys the yeast. There are also actual physical barriers, such as the mucous lining of the digestive tract, which (when in a good state of health) prevents intrusion by yeast or any other undesirable elements. All mucous membranes contain further protective substances which can destroy invading particles of yeast. I will consider these defences later, in the search for an understanding of candidiasis.

At this stage we should simply recognize that the body possesses an efficient defence capability which deals with toxins, bacteria and yeast, should any of them intrude into areas in which they present a danger. Problems arise when, because of one of a variety of causes, which will be discussed later, our ability to defend against Candida becomes deficient or weakens. If this happens, the controls which keep the yeast in check would be removed, and it could then more easily spread to areas normally out of bounds. If at the same time the foods that the yeast thrives on happen to be in plentiful supply, we have the recipe for an explosion of Candida activity. This is precisely the combination of factors that has been identified as having become widespread in Western society over the past 25 to 30 years.

The introduction of broad-spectrum antibiotics, the use of the contraceptive pill and the widespread proliferation of steroid medication, have all played their part in Candida's growth. In addition, the increase in the use of sugar and sugar-rich foods has provided the yeast with just the sustenance it loves. This is the unfortunate combination of factors that is the root cause of the problem for many people.

A careful look at the nature of the enemy is necessary, together with consideration of those factors and circumstances which allow it to proliferate, and what the consequences of such a proliferation might be. We will then be in a position to consider methods of controlling Candida. Fortunately this is the brighter side of the sorry mess. For it seems unlikely that the causative elements of the 'yeast explosion' are going to disappear, and so the fact that control is possible, in the majority of cases, is a blessing indeed.

It is important to understand that the conditions listed above are certainly not always the result of Candida infection. It is, however, true that all of these can be partly or entirely a result of candidiasis. It is the view of those practitioners now aware of the possibility of Candida's involvement in common disease problems of this sort that when a combination of such symptoms appears in a person, with no other obvious causes apparent, then Candida should be the prime suspect. Unlike most infection and infestations, it is difficult to test accurately for the presence of Candida to prove or disprove its active presence. This is because, as has already been stated, Candida is present to some extent in all of us, which makes looking for it as pointless as searching for mice in a granary; it is always present, but to what extent? Candida can be cultured in many people's blood, and it is so common in stool cultures that it is usually ignored by microbiologists when they do come across it. Medical researchers have highlighted the difficulty of assessing, purely from tests, whether Candida is active even when it is known to be in an advanced stage of overgrowth.[1]

They report of one group of 48 patients with acute myeloid leukaemia that there was such widespread Candida infiltration in the lungs and other organs that 'entire microscopic fields were filled with mycelia,' and yet the diagnosis could have been assumed from signs without waiting for the time-consuming proof positive from the laboratory. Half of these patients died from candidiasis, and the doctors assert that, had they been able to attack the yeast aggressively earlier, this tragedy may have been averted.

Among the tests discussed were:

1   Faecal culturing of Candida (although the researchers admit this gives 25 per cent false negatives – that is, people of whom it is assumed from this test that they do not have Candida overgrowth, when in fact it is rampantly present).

2   Looking for any rise in the bloodstream of Candida antibodies even within supposedly 'normal' levels (10 per cent false negatives).

3   Pain behind the sternum (breastbone) or thrush in the mouth. These signs are absent in 50 per cent and 30 per cent of patients who die of candidiasis, respectively, showing that their absence proves nothing in terms of whether or not Candida is active. If present, together with other general signs (*see pages 33–4*) they are a strong indication of systemic candidiasis.

4   A low continuous fever for four days or more which fails to respond to antibiotic therapy. In 16 patients with this sign, treated for candidiasis, 11 became free of fever rapidly.

While these signs and assessment methods criteria may be useful in a hospital setting, in private practice or in self-assessment of candidiasis it is generally recognized that the history and present symptoms (as outlined in Chapter 4) give an accurate guide as to whether or not Candida is presently active. The way to prove that a condition (or a cluster of conditions occurring together) is the result of Candida, is to treat it; if the symptoms then disappear the proof is difficult to contest.

Candidiasis is one of the very few instances where the treatment of a health problem is in fact the main means of diagnosis. The initial suspicions that result in the treatment being started, rely upon recognition of the sort of symptoms that suggest the presence of Candida, as well as an awareness of those factors that influence Candida's development and behaviour.

A careful background history which looks at previous and current medical treatment and drug usage, as well as at diet and stress factors, will give clear indications as to the likelihood, or otherwise, of Candida being a possible culprit.

It is these areas that we are going to explore, in order to formulate a series of recommendations for the control of Candida, and for the prevention of its accompanying complications.

The potentially disastrous health damage caused by the exaggerated activity of a once fairly harmless interaction between ourselves and a yeast that is usually easily tolerated and controlled, is one of the complications of civilization. Candidiasis is rapidly becoming so widespread as to constitute an epidemic. The failure, thus far, by all but a handful of doctors to recognize the situation is tragic, for the degree of human suffering involved is enormous. Prevention is not difficult, and control, while a slow process (taking months, not years), is not beyond the limits of any intelligent person.

The major credit for the unravelling of this mystery belongs to one man, who recognized that what he was seeing in his own patients had world-wide importance. He first set about diligently assembling his evidence, which he presented in a scientific journal.[2] He then went back to his task of investigation. Over a period of years his excellent clinical results in treating an enormous range of diseases, from acne to schizophrenia, and what appeared to be multiple sclerosis, were so impressive that in true fashion the world began to beat a path to his door. Dr C. Orion Truss, of Birmingham, Alabama, will be remembered for his work in this field by hundreds of thousands of grateful people. His masterly investigation and research, conducted in a normal medical practice, shows how important simple observation is in the quest for knowledge and the understanding of humanity's ills. Dr Truss has written his own history of this research, and of the whole story of Candida, in his book *The Missing Diagnosis.*

That book, and the excellent book on the same subject by another renowned American practitioner, Dr William Crook, entitled *The Yeast Connection*, both suggest for their attack on yeast the use of an antifungal drug called nystatin. They also suggest other methods, including nutrition and desensitization. This book, however, will not attempt to echo the drug approach suggested by these two practitioners, but will present non-drug alternatives to the use of nystatin. This is not to say that nystatin and other antifungal drugs should never be used, only that in most cases there are other, apparently safer ways of restoring the competence of the body to fight the yeast itself. There are sound reasons for trying to find anti-candida alternatives (as will be explained in later chapters), including many naturally occurring nutrients which enhance the controlling of the wildly prolif-erating yeast without producing resistant strains, something now thought likely when nystatin is used for long periods. This is the only reason this book has needed to be written, for in every other way the two books mentioned above are excellent and valuable contributions to the literature of health.

We need now to take a closer look at the nature of the enemy, what makes it active and how to recognize such activity. After that we will begin to learn how to deal with it.

Chapter 2

CANDIDA AND
YOUR DEFENCE SYSTEM

Candida albicans is a member of the yeast family. Strictly speaking it is a member of a sub-group of that family of organisms known as fungi (or moulds). Yeasts live practically everywhere on the planet and can derive their nutrients from most organic sources. This means anything that is alive, or has been alive, can support yeasts. Rather than having roots like other plants, yeasts can derive their nutrients via the enzymes which they produce. Given the right conditions for growth and replication, yeast is capable of almost explosive growth, as anyone who has made bread will testify.

Roger Williams, a world-renowned research scientist, states that if a single yeast cell is given a highly favourable environment, with a good assortment of nutrients, and the correct temperature, it can, within 24 hours, produce a colony of over 100 yeast cells. At this rate of reproduction, Williams calculates, within one week, one cell could turn into a yeast colony weighing one billion tons.[1] The fact that this has not happened, and that it is not likely to happen, is solely because the environment is seldom ideal for any creature on earth, least of all for yeast. It does, however, highlight a very pertinent point in our understanding of the Candida problem: Candida is a yeast which lives inside you and me and, as far as is known, every other adult on earth, and most children as well. It seldom takes over our entire body, but when it does the consequences are horrific. It can only achieve such a state if the environment for it is excellent, and if the defence mechanisms that the body has with which to control its spread are weakened or absent.

As Williams points out, in nature yeast cells are almost always hampered by imperfect or inadequate environmental conditions. Were it not so, they would have engulfed the earth long ago. Just the same fact controls the colonies of Candida (and other yeasts) that live in and on you and me.

Uninvited Residents of the Body

Candida is usually a resident of the digestive system, largely in the intestines. It also tends to occupy sites in the vaginal regions and on the skin.

Research has shown that almost everyone has antibodies to Candida. When such antibodies are found this indicates that the individual's immune system has been challenged to respond to the presence of the yeast. Dr Truss states that by the age of six months, at the latest, Candida is living in or on at least 90 per cent of people, as evidenced by a positive skin test reaction when extracts of Candida are injected just under the skin.[2] This reaction shows that there has been a previous presence of the yeast to which the body has developed defensive antibodies.

The fact that it is in all of us, and yet many people sail through life with no apparent ill effects, indicates that we have learned to cope with our uninvited yeast passengers. Unlike certain other minute creatures that live in our digestive tract, and which serve a useful purpose, such as Lactobacillus acidophilus (which helps with the breakdown of our foodstuff and helps in the synthesis of some of the B vitamins), there is no symbiotic relationship with Candida. There is no 'trade-off' whereby houseroom is given in exchange for some useful function. So Candida is a pure and simple parasite – a freeloader. This is perhaps inevitable, in terms of the multitude of opportunistic microscopic creatures in both the animal and vegetable kingdom. Most, if not all, plants and animals enjoy similar relationships with bacteria and fungi. Some of these relationships are mutually beneficial and some are distinctly one-sided. So Candida, for all the musicality of its name, is an unwelcome boarder and a potential danger throughout life. Once we know just what sort of situations will remove our ability to control it naturally, and what will give it that extra capacity to proliferate by virtue of an environment conducive to its growth, we will begin to understand what needs to be done to contain it when it gets out of hand and starts producing health problems.

Part of the solution involves coming to an understanding of the ways in which the body has learned to take care of the threat of parasites. It may be that we cannot actually stop it from taking up squatters' rights in the body, but we can certainly confine its activities to a small and relatively safe part of the premises.

The Way the Body Defends Itself

We need to understand some aspects of the body's amazing defensive capability. It has long been observed that people who survive certain infections seldom suffer from that same disease again. They develop antibodies to the infecting organism. Apart from conferring such specific resistance to various disease-causing micro-organisms, the immune system plays a vital role in other biological reactions. In relation to infection we have, in essence, two systems of defence. One is based on the thymus gland (which lies just below the breast bone), which produces what are called T-cells.

Another part of the immune system is made up of different types of white blood cells, called B-cells. These protect you from most bacterial invaders, and some viral infections. By producing molecules called antibodies, the B-cells neutralize many potential enemies. The two systems, together making up the surveillance and protection agency of the body, work in harmony – the thymus, it is thought, takes the leading role.[3]

The Body's Front-line Defenders

The white blood cells, which act as the soldiers in the front line of the battle, are manufactured mainly in the marrow of the long bones of the body. Some of these actually are turned into T-cells, by the influence of hormones from the thymus gland. Other white blood cells are turned into what are called lymphocytes. Anything that tries to get into the bloodstream, or the interior of the body, has to contend with the T- and B-cells, and their powerful ability to neutralize foreign substances or organisms. If a B-cell senses a foreign organism, it produces antibodies that are specific against the invader. At the same time, other B-cells are alerted to the alien presence, which causes them to manufacture antibodies to destroy the enemy.

It is believed that there are in excess of a million different kinds of antibodies in the bloodstream. As they are manufactured and deployed against the intruder, the lymphocytes go into action, with other white blood cells, to dispose of the debris and waste products of the battle between the intruder and the body. Thus a condition such as influenza is self-limiting, in that the fever and the symptoms of aching represent the intense activity that is going on in the body to deal with the invading virus, as well as the effects of the resulting toxicity of the breakdown products of the battle.

When T-cells come across an invading organism, whether this

be a virus or a fungus such as Candida (or even a mutant cancer cell), they produce what are called lymphokines which can kill micro-organisms (or cancer cells). One such lymphokine which has received much attention is interferon. Lymphokines can also call up assistance from powerful allies in this battle called macrophages, which can eliminate micro-organisms and tumour cells by literally swallowing them whole. Sometimes the T-cells act as 'helper' cells to the B-cells in their production of antibodies to fight the invader. They can also act as what are called 'suppressor' cells, to stop a defensive process from getting out of hand, when there may be a danger of B- or T-cells actually attacking friendly tissues in the body.

What If the Immune System Is Inefficient?

When for any one of a number of reasons (which we will consider in a later chapter) the immune system becomes weakened, we talk of the person being immuno-deficient, or of having a poor immune response. It is when these valiant soldiers – the T- and B-cells – and the macrophages and their various assistants are put into a weakened state that silent 'squatters' in the body can become free of the constraints that the defence system normally imposes and spread to areas beyond their normal territory. At that point a vast array of problems and symptoms can arise.

This system of defence, with its checks and balances, may become disrupted to such an extent that the condition, now known simply by the initials AIDS, may occur. The initials stand for Acquired Immuno-Deficiency Syndrome, and in this condition it is the T-cells (from the thymus gland) that function inadequately. In fact the ratio between the helper and suppressor cells alters so that there is an excess of suppressor cells, in contrast with the situation that exists in normal health. Much research in the treatment of immune-related conditions focuses on methods which can enhance the function of the thymus gland so that it can produce a balanced and adequate supply of active T-cells. Among the nutrient factors which we can use to this end are vitamin C and the amino acid arginine. The amounts used in treating conditions, such as AIDS, where the immune system is severely disrupted are very large indeed (upwards of 20 g of vitamin C daily, and 3–5 g of arginine).

When the immune system is in a weakened state, not only do infections become more frequent but severe consequences arise, such as a greater likelihood of cancer developing, because of the reduced surveillance by the B- and T-cells. In such a condition of inadequate protection it is no wonder that the ever-present opportunistic yeast may slip through the defence barrier and advance to areas previously closed to it. This is a simplistic picture of what happens, but it contains the essential facts.

Some Consequences of Yeast Overgrowth

It is known that before it becomes invasive the yeast (Candida) alters to a different form, known as its mycelial fungal form, in which it has characteristics which make it more dangerous – such as a root structure enabling it to penetrate through the mucosal barriers, for example that of the digestive tract, with a variety of harmful consequences resulting from such easy access of toxins and the breakdown products of digestion directly into the bloodstream (*see Chapter 4*).

Research by Dr Truss[1] indicates that many of the toxic effects noted with Candida activity result from its ability to manufacture, under appropriate conditions, the substance acetaldehyde. He points out that this well-known toxin could produce both the clinical and the laboratory characteristics of Candida infection. He has analysed the amino acid profiles of affected individuals in order to arrive at his finding, and maintains that this theory appeals because it defines the symptoms of chronic yeast infection in terms of a toxin which common strains of Candida can be shown to produce in laboratory conditions. This provides the chemical link between normal yeast fermentation and the metabolic abnormalities found in susceptible patients. Dr Truss stresses that it is highly probable that the symptoms experienced by many Candida sufferers relate directly to the ability of yeast to ferment sugar into acetaldehyde in the body. There are now tests which take advantage of this and which measure any rise in blood alcohol levels after a 'sugar loading' in which alcohol (such as acetaldehyde) is measured after the taking of a specific amount of sugar on an empty stomach. This 'gut fermentation' test is not foolproof for a number of reasons, including the fact that other organisms, including certain bacteria which can live in the gut, can ferment sugar.

Some laboratory technicians performing these tests (and many practitioners involved in treating chronic candidiasis) report being able to smell the alcohol resulting from eating sugar in people who never drink alcohol at all. In my personal practice I have treated individuals for candidiasis who have been breathalysed and found to be over the legal limit of alcohol in their bloodstream, despite their not having consumed any alcohol.

Amalgam Fillings and Immune Suppression

There is also evidence from a variety of sources[3] that there is a degree of immune system depression which results from mercury toxicity reaching the body via amalgam fillings in the teeth. A number of researchers have shown there are several ways in which this highly toxic metal is able to penetrate the body, and that this has a specific harmful effect on the immune system. There is evidence that this can be linked with the spread of

Candida activity. A number of dentists are now helping affected individuals by removing mercury amalgams and replacing them with either a composite or gold filling. It should be stressed that research into the relationship between mercury, derived from amalgam fillings, and health problems in general and Candida involvement in particular is as yet incomplete. That there is a link seems probable, however, and it is worth considering alternative choices for fillings other than amalgams which contain mercury.

The replacement of existing fillings may be required in cases where a link can be demonstrated between a person's health and measurable mercury toxicity resulting from amalgams. The use of supplemental amino acid compounds, such as Glutathione, and of vitamin C, can help to ease mercury deposits from the body. Tests can be done to measure the sensitivity of the body to mercury, and also to measure the levels of mercury in the mouth (escaping as a gas), as well as the electrical activity in the teeth, set up by the combinations of metals in the mouth. These methods, as well as measuring mercury levels via hair analysis, can all indicate just how pronounced this problem is in any particular individual.

Denture Hygiene and Yeast

A further dental hazard related to candidiasis was discovered in a study which looked at 50 consecutive patients with respiratory disease who had all developed candidiasis in the mouth and pharynx. Dentures were found to be worn by 32 of those in the study, and this was thought to be a major predisposing factor in their Candida onset (among the others were the use of cortisone, antibiotics and immune-suppressing sedatives). The researchers stated, 'Dentures cause tissue trauma, provide sites for [yeast] colonization and diminish salivary flow. Saliva is necessary for normal oral immune defence.'[6]

It was found that if dentures were treated with antifungal

15

chemicals this helped prevent this hazard. Regular sterilizing of dentures is suggested as a safe preventive measure, along with oral rinsing with dilute Aloe vera juice (an antifungal substance – *see pages 61–2*).

Yeast Control Objectives

Our ultimate attempt to neutralize and control the spread and effects of Candida (for we can seldom get rid of it completely) depends upon the use of whatever safe methods we have at our disposal to deprive it of its ideal nutrients, while at the same time building up and enhancing the depleted immune system. The immune system can then get on with the job of keeping Candida in check. It is this double thrust of activity which we must undertake if we are to do more than temporarily suppress Candida. The use of an antifungal drug will, it is true, in time destroy a great deal of Candida's potency and reduce its resultant symptoms. However, this recuperative process will stop the moment the drug is no longer taken.

The answer to controlling Candida in the long term lies in a multi-pronged attack which simultaneously:

1 deprives the yeast of its optimum nutrient environment ('starve the yeast')

2 actively kills yeast using safe non-toxic methods

3 actively focuses on restoring the body's normal controls over yeast, by supporting the immune system and encouraging a healthy intestinal flora

4 helps to restore damaged tissues, such as the mucous membrane of the digestive tract.

16

As we will see, there are other methods which, it is thought, can help by altering the ability of the yeast to multiply. We will consider these natural, safe alternatives to the use of drugs later.

What about Antifungal Drugs?

It must, however, be stated that there are conditions in which the use of antifungal drugs is to be advocated, especially if the condition is such as to indicate that the process of recovery is going to be a very long one. In the main, however, once we can learn to recognize the symptoms that indicate Candida getting out of hand, the natural, non-drug methods that I suggest will work, and work well.

Nystatin is the main such antifungal drug now in use. While effective against certain Candida strains, others are resistant to it. Not being a broad-spectrum antifungal agent, it allows proliferation of other fungi, such as trichophyton, when Candida is attacked.[7] An alternative exists in caprylic acid, an extract of coconuts (*see pages 66–7*). The use of antifungal drugs is discussed more fully in Chapter 5.

None of these drugs is usually used with a comprehensive antifungal dietary and supplement approach which would encourage a healthier digestive tract and immune system.

Drugs are seldom necessary at all, since the methods which will be outlined in later chapters are safer and of proven efficacy.

Reminder

Let us not lose sight of the fact that Candida lives in every one of us and that it usually produces no symptoms unless the environment in which it lives (our body) has been compromised.

Diagnosis of yeast involvement in health problems is not a case of establishing whether or not yeast is present because it always is, to some extent. Rather it is the task of the health care provider who is advising anyone with yeast-related problems to attempt to discover what underlying factors have allowed yeast to proliferate and to focus attention on these – as well as to control fungal activity.

Any approach which targets the yeast alone will result in a return of symptoms sooner rather than later. It is not just the yeast which we need to control, but the causes which have allowed it to opportunistically explode into action.

We will now go on to consider just what can happen to weaken your wonderful defence mechanism, the immune system, as well as additional ways in which Candida is sometimes allowed to go on the rampage, and so begin to infest other areas of your body.

Chapter 3

HOW CANDIDA
GETS OUT OF HAND

There are a number of predisposing factors which allow Candida to get wildly out of control. To a greater or lesser extent these same factors may be involved in the more subtle spread of Candida, which represents what happens in the majority of people affected by the sort of symptoms outlined in Chapter 1.

Anyone affected by yeast overgrowth is likely to be able to identify a number of interacting 'causes'. Seldom will only one factor be involved. Among the main ones are:

1   an underlying inherited or acquired deficiency of the immune system

2   the aftermath of steroids (hormones) in food (residues found in factory-farmed meat and poultry, for example) or as medication (cortisone, 'the Pill', etc.)

3   the long-term effects of antibiotics in food (factory-farmed animals or their products, such as milk) or as medication

4   diabetes

5   a diet rich in simple sugars.

As we shall see, these factors are also vitally interconnected with the diet of the individual, which 'feeds' the yeast. We will look at each of these and see how they transform Candida from its relatively docile state into that of a predator. First let us consider ways in which the immune system can be weakened.

Immune System Deficiency

As we have seen in the previous chapter, part of the body's response to an intruder such as Candida is the production of antibodies to meet the particular antigen (a substance which stimulates a response on the part of the immune system) that is present in the foreign substance or organism. Candida has many antigens, and the efficiency with which the defensive operation is carried out against any particular one of these antigens can to some extent be inborn (that is, genetic). There is a great variation in the degree of response in any one person to the different antigens. This can lead to a situation in which the immune system, unable to counteract and expel the Candida invasion adequately, tolerates it in increasing amounts.

Biochemical Individuality

It has been demonstrated by research that we are all bio-chemically unique.[1]

This means that there are wide variations in the particular requirements for any of the over 40 nutrients that we require for survival and health. Many of these individual needs are determined before birth, and this has led to the genetotrophic theory of disease causation. This, put simply, says that because a person has individual inborn requirements, which may vary greatly from a mythical 'average' or 'normal' amount, there is a good chance of one or other of these needs not being met by the normal dietary intake. This leads at best to a lowered degree of function, at worst to a deficiency disease.

To a large extent this individual inborn (genetic) factor also applies to our ability to handle one or other of the pathogens, or micro-organisms, capable of infecting us. This is the case in our ability to handle Candida efficiently. It seems that since infestation by this yeast is almost universal, we are incapable of totally controlling its presence in our bodies. Some people will be more able than others to keep it under control, and limit its spread. Thus some people will, without the involvement of such factors as antibiotics and steroid drugs (*see below*), become 'tolerant' of a degree of spread of the yeast.

The commonest areas for this spread to occur are in the mouth, the throat and in the vaginal areas. If this initially produces a degree of reaction and activity on behalf of the immune system, then we would see manifestations of the condition called thrush. This would flare up periodically when, perhaps, there were factors which lowered the body's general vitality. Eventually, in many cases, the condition might no longer evoke an acute flare-up, but would remain in a semi- permanent, chronic state. This happens when the body becomes 'tolerant' of the yeast's 'foothold' and is no longer able to mount attacks on it. This is an indication of impaired or deficient immune function. Among the many aspects of our environment which can influence this are stress factors, nutritional inadequacy and pollution, as well as the use of specific drugs which weaken the immune system further.

Drugs and Immune Function

We are all nowadays familiar with the concept of tissue and organ transplantation. This involves the use of powerful drugs which are designed to prevent the body of the recipient from rejecting the new foreign tissue or organ. These are called immuno-suppressive drugs, simply because it is their prime task to stop the natural defences from working adequately – in other words, to suppress the immune system. The risk of infection and of other diseases resulting from this is all too familiar to patients who have gone through such treatment. Drugs such as steroids (hormones) have this effect, and these are employed in a variety of conditions ranging from rheumatic disorders to asthma and hormonal imbalances. The most widespread use of steroids, however, is not in the treatment of disease but in the contraceptive pill. One of the most devastating effects of the long-term use of this type of medication is on the immune system in general, and on the ability of Candida to proliferate wildly, in particular. The contraceptive pill is dealt with more fully below.

Immune System Nutrient Support

There are now known to be a variety of nutrient substances which are absolutely vital for the adequate functioning of the immune system.[2]

These include a number of vitamin and mineral substances which have antioxidant properties. This means that they are able to slow down, or stop, a process in which substances known as 'free radicals' can cause tissue damage. The major free-radical scavengers are vitamin C and vitamin E (acting in conjunction with a substance called selenium), as well as certain amino acids (parts of the protein chain) such as methionine, cysteine and glutathione (which is itself a combination of three amino acids: cysteine, glutamic acid and glycine).

Vitamin B_6 (pyridoxine), zinc, manganese and other important nutrients have been shown to be involved in compromising the immune system when the body does not get enough of them.[3]

It should be realized that, apart from the nutrients mentioned in this section, it is possible for any of the 40-plus nutrients vital to life to be required in extraordinary amounts by a particular person to meet idiosyncratic inborn needs. These needs may also vary markedly under different conditions (infection, stress, pregnancy, etc.) in the same person, and so any vitamin, mineral or other nutrient is capable of upsetting the chain of complex biochemical interactions which allow the immune function to operate efficiently. The ones cited above just happen to have a more dramatic impact than some of the others. Assessment of personal needs is a task requiring patience.

Stress and Immune Function

Stress, which involves repeated, or constant, states of anxiety, and all that this entails in terms of depletion of vital nutrient reserves, as well as imbalances of internal secretions and functions, is a major cause of immune incompetence.

A new scientific discipline has emerged called psycho-neuroimmunology, which studies the direct connection between our emotions and how efficiently, or otherwise, our immune system behaves. The evidence is that there is a very clear link between the mind and the body operating through the defence system, which is meant to protect both. One of the ways in which this can be most dramatically demonstrated is that during periods of stress (students during exam time, for example) people become far more prone to infection. This indicates the lowered efficiency of their immune system, as well as the increased usage by the body of vital nutrients such as zinc and vitamin C at such times.

The interaction between anxiety/stress conditions and

nutritional imbalances leads to the immune system being deprived of the ability to operate efficiently. If at the same time there is increased demand on the effective functioning of the immune system, to meet environmental or nutritional toxicity (pollution of air, cigarette smoke, alcohol, caffeine-rich drinks such as coffee, chocolate and tea) then a complex picture emerges in which excessive demands, inadequate nutrition (with associated deficiencies) and perhaps drug usage, such as the contraceptive pill, all interact to deplete the immune function. Let us examine the manner in which drugs in common use can further complicate the situation.

Antibiotics, 'the Pill' and Steroids

It is clear from many years of research that the use of antibiotics removes from the scene biological controls over the yeast that lives in us. As has been mentioned, one of the major sites for this to take place is the long, dark, warm and moist (ideal environment for yeast) digestive tract, which it should be noted is also inhabited by upwards of 5 lb of other micro-organisms, most of which are friendly and helpful to the body. One such friend is *Lactobacillus acidophilus*, which by its presence helps to keep a check on the spread of yeast. When antibiotics are used to destroy pathogenic (harmful) micro-organisms which might be harming the body (as in treating an infection), the friendly bacteria in the bowel are also destroyed, or severely damaged. When this occurs, the yeast, which is totally unaffected by the antibiotic (being a yeast and not bacteria), will find room for expansion. This becomes even more likely as the resistance of the immune system will at that time be compromised. In a variety of ways the same thing happens with the use of steroid drugs, such as cortisone (even cortisone ointments, so commonly prescribed for skin problems, cause a yeast increase by being absorbed into

24

the system). All steroids, including those used in the contra-ceptive pill, will have a depressing effect on the immune system.

Food Sources of These Drugs

It is worth noting at this point that there is another, almost totally ignored source of antibiotics and hormonal residues, to which all but the vegan sector of the population are exposed. This is of course the eating of commercially reared meat (with the exception of lamb) and poultry (and eggs). Antibiotics and hormones are fed to animals in order to speed their growth as well as to control the heightened susceptibility to disease that their unnatural existence generates.

Anyone who has been regularly eating beef, pork, veal and chicken (and many people eat one or more of these daily) will have absorbed prodigious amounts of antibiotic and hormone residues (unless the source of the meat was from a farm which did not employ the addition of such drugs).

Unfortunately, antibiotic residues also find their way into dairy produce (including eggs), unless this is of guaranteed organic origin, so even vegetarians are likely to be affected by antibiotics in their food.

Low-level intake of these substances over many years may have a devastating effect on the ability to control Candida, as would the regular employment of these drugs in the form of medications. This area is yet to be adequately researched, but it does provide one more argument in favour of adopting a vegetarian diet, low in dairy produce.

It has also been noted that, because of the hormonal changes that take place during pregnancy, a degree of control over Candida is lost. Yeast therefore finds this a good time to expand its activities.

Twentieth-century Young Woman

Most people with Candida problems are women, and most are under 50 years of age. Why?

Imagine if you will a young woman who has grown up in this era characterized by common usage of these drugs – antibiotics and steroid medication. She has had antibiotics prescribed to her over the years for minor problems such as tonsillitis and ear infection. She may have then developed cystitis from time to time, and also have had a broad-spectrum antibiotic for this. Her skin may have had a good deal of acne, and again this would commonly have been attacked with antibiotics. Should she have had cause, she may have had steroids for asthma or some other condition. Going on 'the Pill', and subsequently coming off it and becoming pregnant, would also have enhanced the chances of yeast spreading, and would have caused further problems (the acne and cystitis are frequent examples of Candida activity). Thus the child in her womb would be exposed to a variety of antigens (up to 790) from the Candida activity in her body, all the while inheriting the possibility of a weak immune response (not all children inherit a weak response). Thus the pattern will be set to repeat itself. We have still left out of this picture all the other variables, such as nutritional imbalances, which are common in modern society; pollution; excessive use of sugar-rich foods (which yeast loves); and stress factors in general. The picture emerges of a person who is doing just about all that is possible to bring about the ideal conditions for yeast to thrive in.

The result, in terms of the general population, of this typical scenario? An explosion of Candida-caused problems, over the past 30 years or so, which is now reaching epidemic proportions.

We will discuss later a very important aspect of Candida's spread, which is the diet of the individual, not in the sense of helping to create a situation in which the immune system is less efficient, but as adding actual supporting nutrients to Candida.

The two main areas in which this occurs are the use of sugar-rich foods, which all yeasts love, as well as foods that are themselves associated with yeasts or fungi. In the mean time it should be evident that many aspects of life in 'civilized' society are working to the disadvantage of our defensive ability, and to the advantage of prospective enemies, such as Candida.

Dr Truss' Views

Dr Truss, who has done so much to research and publicize the Candida problem, is scathing in his attack on the use of certain drugs which have compounded the problem. Antibiotics are often used inadvisedly, in cases in which they have no role to play at all. Incorrectly diagnosed viral and fungal conditions may be uselessly treated by antibiotics, for example. This actually increases the likelihood of the condition worsening. The treatment of acne with tetracycline is another major cause of Candida spreading, and Truss insists that there is no way anyone suffering from Candida problems can control the condition if he or she continues with tetracycline. In many cases acne is actually the direct result of Candida infection, and will worsen rather than improve on such treatment.

In the use of the contraceptive hormone, too, Truss sees great harm. Fully 35 per cent of women using the Pill have, associated with it, acute vaginal candidiasis. There are undoubtedly many others who have less pronounced changes in this regard, as their immune competence is gradually compromised by the hormonal onslaught. As Truss points out, 'Chronic yeast vaginitis tends to be at its worst when progesterone levels are high, as in pregnancy, and the luteal phase of the menstrual cycle. Therefore the progesterone component of contraceptive hormones may well be responsible for their effect.'

It is clear that the association between Candida vaginitis and emotional problems such as irritability and depression frequently appears soon after the first use of the contraceptive pill. It is worth reflecting on the fact that the degree of biological individuality which we display in our individual reactions to any harmful factor such as Candida must play a large part in deciding just who will, and who will not, succumb to a spread of Candida. Since 35 per cent of women do not control the vaginal Candida when on the Pill, we must assume that the other 65 per cent do. This highlights the fact that for many people there is an inborn genetic weakness in their ability to meet such a challenge. For some this will have been acquired via the very factors we have been discussing in this chapter: antibiotics, immune system weakened by stress, nutritional factors, etc. We shall see that the approach to controlling Candida must include methods that deal both with the building up of the immune system as well as with reducing as many factors as possible which help to assist the yeast in its advance. Among the most important of these is the elimination of the use (unless absolutely vital) of antibiotics, hormone preparations and contraceptive pills, as well as altering the diet to avoid actually feeding the yeast.

Since yeast loves sugar, it is clear that if a person has additional levels of sugar in the bloodstream, as in a diabetic condition, this will fuel the spread of Candida. For this reason diabetic individuals are more prone than average to Candida problems, and they must be even more rigorous in their efforts to control it.

The possible involvement of mercury toxicity in harming the immune system's control of Candida has been mentioned (*see pages 14–15*) and deserves re-emphasis.

Foods that Help to Spread Candida

Yeast loves carbohydrate-rich foods. This in effect means that we must attempt to deprive it of its sustenance by limiting, or cutting out all together, all sugar-rich foods and refined carbohydrates.

Details of this will be outlined in the nutritional programme (*see Chapter 7*).

It is also considered by many experts to be important that the intake of any foods that contain fermented products, moulds or fungi be limited.[1]

Many anti-Candida programmes make a great effort to emphasize this restriction ('no yeast-based or fermented foods!'). The reasons for such restrictions, however, are not always explained or even logical.

First it must be clearly understood that avoiding such foods is necessary only if the person with a Candida problem has become sensitized – and therefore allergic or sensitive to – fungus-related substances. If not there is no reason to add yet another restriction to an already somewhat complex programme.

How Can You Know Whether it Is Necessary or Not?

A simple exclusion period of 10 to 14 days, during which all yeast-based foods are eliminated, is a basic method. During this time there is a need to keep a careful 'symptom' score (*see Chapter 7*) which will set the scene for a definitive experiment. After the period of yeast-food elimination (it takes at least five days for all traces of the excluded food to be cleared by the system) you can introduce a 'challenge' in which you eat a small amount of a yeast-based food (or a fragment of a yeast tablet) twice in one day, and observe any reactions.

Did your symptoms improve when not eating such foods?

Did they return when you reintroduced these foods?

A 'Yes' answer to either question suggests that you should investigate further and that you would probably benefit from leaving such foods out of your diet for a while.

The foods that are most suspect if yeast is not well tolerated include vinegar, alcoholic beverages, yeast extracts and spreads, mushrooms, blue cheeses, and anything with a mould on it. This list is given more fully in Chapter 6. Once Candida is controlled, unless a yeast sensitivity or allergy exists, there is no reason to keep to a strict prohibition, but the return of classic symptoms of Candida activity, such as abdominal bloating after eating one of the offending foods, will tell you if it is time to return for a period to the avoidance strategy.

Just as foods which contain moulds or fungi are considered undesirable, it may be found that symptoms are worse in humid, damp environments, which are conducive to mould and fungus spores being present in the atmosphere. Thus, it is important to eliminate from the home any areas of damp (on walls, etc.).

An Anti-Candida Programme Is Not Forever!

Candida gets out of hand because we allow it to. We may well do so in ignorance, but it is folly to blame the yeast when we have the power to control it, as millions of people have done before. Once you begin to suspect that your many and varied symptoms (*see Chapter 4*) may be the result of Candida activity, it is time to grasp the problem firmly and take responsibility for the situation. Candida will not go away on its own. Its current spree may be the result of any combination of factors which have released it from the body's normal efficient control. To get it back where it belongs (or at least to where it can do least harm) we must restore our defence capacity to its optimum, and we must stop doing those things that are helping the yeast to thrive. It's as simple as that. You can do this by your own efforts, by the reform of your dietary pattern, by the use of particular nutrient substances, and by reducing the overall levels of stress and pollution in your immediate environment. Once you have put Candida in its place, you can relax your vigilance to a great extent, in the sense of allowing your diet to contain certain of the 'undesirable' substances from time to time, but you should be aware of the factors which allow Candida to advance in the first place, and avoid these as stringently as possible.

We will now look at the sort of problems that Candida can cause when it gets out of control. Be prepared for some surprises.

Chapter 4

CANDIDA
AND ITS CONSEQUENCES
TO YOUR HEALTH

The actual list of conditions in which Candida has been implicated as a major causative factor is very long indeed.

There are dozens of health problems which are yeast related, some minor such as dandruff, but many which are disabling in their severity.

Just How Widespread Are
Such Candida-related Health Problems?

According to activist author Gill Jacobs, fully a third of the populations of Western industrialized countries have illnesses which are linked to Candida, which means hundreds of millions of people.

As has been mentioned, it is necessary to deduce the involvement of Candida from the history of the patient. (Were antibiotics used? Is, or was, the contraceptive pill in use? Have cortisone or other steroids, e.g. prednisone, been employed? etc.)

The range and type of symptoms also give indications of Candida's involvement. This is because it is virtually useless asking a microbiology lab to look for Candida's presence, since we already know it to be present in practically all adults and most children within the first few months of life. So what would an analysis prove? We can usually conclude from the history and the symptoms that Candida seems to be involved. The proof of its involvement is obtained by carrying out an anti-Candida programme and finding out whether or not this gets rid of most of the symptoms.

Before considering them all (or at least the major ones) one by one, let us look at a list of the sort of conditions that are now known to be the possible result of Candida's activity:

- vaginitis
- thrush (oral or vaginal)
- endometriosis (disorder involving the lining of the uterus)
- athlete's foot
- acne
- dandruff
- headaches (migraine type)
- fatigue
- constipation
- bloating
- allergy
- sensitivity to perfumes, fumes, chemical odours
  and tobacco smoke
- poor memory, feelings of unreality, irritability, inability
  to concentrate
- depression
- numbness, tingling and weak muscles
- painful muscles
- heartburn
- abdominal pain
- diarrhoea
- Irritable Bowel Syndrome

- premenstrual tension
- recurrent sore throats and nasal congestion
- recurrent ear infections
- swelling and discomfort in joints
- blurred vision
- and so on.

The diagnosis becomes more clear if symptoms are aggravated during damp weather (or in damp places) or when in an environment with a lot of mould or fungus. If the symptoms are worse after eating sugar-rich or fungus-containing foods, the evidence for Candida's involvement becomes stronger.

Local Candida Symptoms
Start Before General Ones

After we have looked at some of these conditions more closely, we will try to pull the key information together in the form of a questionnaire, which should enable you to assess the chances of Candida being involved in your health make-up. Truss draws a picture of a typical case of chronic Candida infection in his article 'Restoration of Immunological Competence to Candida Albicans'.[1]

He states, after pointing to the influence of multiple pregnancies, birth-control pills, antibiotics and cortisone, as well as other factors that depress the immune system:

> *The onset of local symptoms of yeast infection, in relation to the use of these drugs, is especially significant and usually precedes the systemic response. Repeated courses of antibiotics and birth-control pills, often punctuated with multiple pregnancies, lead to ever increasing symptoms of mucosal infections in the vagina and gastro-intestinal tract. Accompanying these are manifestations of*

tissue injury, based on immunological and possibly toxic responses to yeast products released into the systemic circulation. Many infections are secondary to allergic responses of the mucous membranes of the respiratory tract, urethra and bladder, necessitating increasingly frequent antibiotic therapy that simultaneously aggravates, and perpetuates, the underlying cause of the allergic membrane, that allowed the infection. Depression is common, often associated with difficulty in memory, reasoning and concentration. These symptoms are especially severe in women, who in addition have great difficulty with the explosive irritability, crying and loss of self-confidence that are so characteristic of abnormal function of the ovarian hormones.

Women – The Main Candida Target

Truss then points out that accompanying this sad catalogue are what he calls 'poor end-organ response' resulting in acne; loss of libido (disinterest in sex); menstrual bleeding and cramps; intolerance to foods and chemicals, etc. The commonest (but by no means only) type of individual suffering from Candida infection, is seen to be a woman somewhere between puberty and the menopause who has undergone some, or all, of the predisposing factors described previously, and who has some, or all, of the symptoms outlined in Truss' picture above. A mixture of unaccountable vaginal and bowel symptoms, ranging from discharge and itching to bloating, discomfort, diarrhoea and/or constipation, as well as an array of mental-emotional symptoms are typical. Classically such women are labelled as neurotic, and this must be the crowning insult to an individual who has literally begun to feel her body and mind giving way in all directions.

Digestive Tract Colonization

The vaginal and intestinal tracts are the most usual areas for Candida to inhabit, since they provide the damp atmosphere and the nutrients it thrives on. If circumstances allow, Candida has been known to spread along the entire length of the digestive tract, from the anus to the mouth. The tongue may be coated, and there may be yeast deposits on the insides of the cheeks, the corners of the mouth and gums. White spots and a coating on the tongue are the obvious signs, accompanied by a soreness and tingling of the gums. When the oesophagus is affected it can result in symptoms commonly assigned to 'heartburn'; indigestion and acid stomach are symptoms which can be the result of Candida activity in the stomach region. If the infestation is prolific in the small or large intestine, then diarrhoea may be the result. This may be chronic and may be accompanied by mucus and/or blood. There may be cramp-like pains ('spastic colon') and colicky pains, often associated with difficulty in passing normal bowel motions. Bloating and distension of the abdomen is a frequent occurrence with Candida, and there may be a variety of abdominal noises as a result. If constipation is indeed a factor, then haemorrhoids are a likely consequence, as is the possibility of rectal discomfort and itching.

What Happens When Candida Becomes a Fungus?

Candida is what is known as a dimorphic organism. This means that it has two quite separate identities and that the very nature of Candida changes under certain conditions. It can turn into what is called its 'mycelial fungal' form from its simple yeast form. In the yeast form it has no root, but in its fungal form it produces what are called *rhizoids*. These are long structures, similar to roots. The complication that this presents is that these 'roots' can actually penetrate through the mucosa (lining) of the tissue in which they are growing. One of the key controls which prevents this change is the abundant presence of the B vitamin, biotin. In good health, biotin is manufactured in the intestines by friendly bacteria. After antibiotic treatment (or anything else which upsets their function) these bacteria may become severely depleted and unable to manufacture biotin. Thus control is removed from the yeast and the aggressive fungal form emerges to start its onslaught on new territories in the body. Supplementation with biotin helps to control this, as does restoration of normal bowel flora ecology via supplements of potent, viable strains of these friendly bacteria. These are important and usually successful strategies in the campaign against Candida. Until this control occurs, the change from yeast to fungus allows a breach by fungal roots of the boundary between the body proper and the self-contained world of the digestive tract. This allows substances to enter the bloodstream which would otherwise have been kept out by this boundary. The fungal form of the Candida organism is invasive, and it can use this avenue to enter the body proper.

The main result of the breaking of the intestinal barrier is that undigested proteins from the food eaten, as well as toxic wastes from the Candida infestation, may begin to circulate in the bloodstream. These are frequently the cause of a wide variety of disseminated symptoms, often of an allergic type.

'Brain Allergies'

If these substances reach the brain, there is a chance for the production of what have been termed 'brain allergies'.[2] These can result in a wide variety of mood and personality problems, ranging from depression, irritability and mood swings to conditions which look for all the world like the symptoms of schizophrenia.

Substances which enter the brain and act upon the receptors there to produce mental and personality symptoms have been given the label *exorphins*.[3] This differentiates them from endorphins, which are substances produced in the body which have roles to play in the functioning of many aspects of the biochemistry of life, including pain control. The externally originating substances (proteins from incompletely digested food, for example) which slip into the bloodstream through the gates opened by fungal 'roots' of Candida are able to cause havoc with whatever tissues they contact. They will be seen as 'foreign' by the immune system, which will attempt to neutralize them. If such a process is long continued – and this sort of thing can run on for many years – then this in itself is a factor contributing to the ultimate depletion of the immune function of the body. It simply becomes overwhelmed by the constant onslaught. The defensive reaction by the immune system to such substances may result in a wide range of what are seen as allergic symptoms, including asthmatic attacks, nasal and respiratory conditions, skin reactions, palpitations, muscle and joint aches and swellings, etc.

Reproductive Organ Dysfunction

The female reproductive organs are a major site for Candida activity. If it irritates the urethra it can be a common cause of cystitis. If, for any of a number of reasons, the acidity of the region alters, then the relatively benign yeast form can alter into the fungal form and become actively invasive and spread to other regions, accessible from the vagina. This can lead to inflammatory conditions in the womb, Fallopian tubes and ovaries themselves (*see Chapter 8*). A wide variety of consequences can be envisaged, including the tragic possibility of infertility or sterility. The symptoms related to Candida involvement in this region can range from frequency of urination, coupled with a burning sensation, to chronic discharge, as well as premenstrual and menstrual problems, and the whole gamut of inflammatory and infectious involvements of the reproductive system.

What about PMT?

An American hospital study[1] strongly supported a link between much PMT and Candida activity. Thirty-two women with severe symptoms of premenstrual syndrome, as well as vaginal candidiasis, were treated with a diet low in yeast and sugars (*see Chapter 6*) together with antifungal medication. They were compared with an equal number of women with similar problems who did not receive the anti-Candida approach. All these patients had previously failed to respond to treatment of their PMT using vitamin treatment and psychotherapy.

The results? Two thirds of the women receiving anti-Candida therapy showed significant PMT relief, while none of those not having this approach improved. The study clearly showed that if PMT and thrush co-exist, dealing with the yeast will often clear the other symptoms as well, thus implicating yeast's activities in much PMT.

Candida, the Mind and the Emotions

The concurrence of mild, or major, emotional and mental symptoms with any such pattern of ill health should alert you to the strong possibility of Candida activity. Often mental symptoms are no more than a general feeling of inability to concentrate, accompanied by memory lapses and feelings of lethargy and exhaustion. They may, however, be far more dramatic, as Truss and others have proved. The first articles on the subject, by Truss, discussed the fact that many conditions are given names or labels simply because they fit into a pattern which is more or less recognizable as being similar to a particular known illness. That is to say, a combination of symptoms which may have no obvious cause is somehow more 'manageable' medically if it is labelled.

Truss initially reported on six cases. Two of these women had been repeatedly diagnosed as 'schizophrenic'. Another woman in this original report was diagnosed previously as having 'multiple sclerosis'. Pointing out that they all recovered on anti-yeast treatment, and that they were all in good health up to 17 years after recovery, he asks the pertinent question, 'Were two of these women really schizophrenic, or was it just that Candida albicans was responsible for brain function so abnormal that highly competent specialists never doubted the diagnosis of schizophrenia?'

He further asks, 'In the third woman, did Candida albicans induce neurological abnormalities sufficiently typical of multiple sclerosis that a competent neurologist would mistakenly diagnose the disease?'

He answers by saying that either the treatment dealt with a yeast infection, which can produce symptoms which mimic these diseases (and many others), or that yeast can actually cause the diseases which are labelled with these names. The indication, after many years of work by Truss and others, is that this is not just a case of remission (which is not uncommon in either schizophrenia or multiple sclerosis) but that Candida induces symptoms similar to those of other illnesses, which may then be wrongly diagnosed and labelled.

Candida and Chronic Fatigue (ME)

Most people with Chronic Fatigue Syndrome (also known as ME, myalgic-encephelomyelitis, as well as Post Viral Fatigue Syndrome) are affected with yeast overgrowth, and in many instances this is the major cause of their condition. It was reading about the way the first edition of this book had changed someone's life that first drew my attention to this fact, for it was following the anti-Candida advice contained in it that was credited, by Sue Finlay, with having made all the difference in her recovery from ME.[3]

She tells of how her doctor, at her insistence, had already prescribed nystatin and that this had taken her from 'being confined to bed, hardly able to stand, tears all day and suicidal' to a point where 'the feeling of being poisoned left me, a little energy returned.' She then states that after some months of variable but gradual improvement:

> *I came on the book,* Candida Albicans: Could Yeast Be Your Problem? *by Leon Chaitow. I changed my diet radically. I cut out sugars and refined carbohydrates. All bread, mushrooms, tea, alcohol, vinegar, coffee, chocolate were dropped. All these foods feed the yeast [see Note below]. I used vitamin supplements to enhance my immune system, olive oil and garlic to attack the yeast and acidophilus powder to replace the Candida with healthy intestinal flora. I ate vegetables, salads, whole cereals and fruit in abundance. At present I am able to walk nearly half a mile without total collapse, I am beginning to work in the garden a little, I still have to rest every day and be careful not to overdo things and cause a relapse, but I have had eight months of improvement and am steadily reducing the nystatin.*

Sue Finlay has continued to improve, and her message is the one I want people with ME to listen to. It is not all in the mind. ME is more likely to cause depression than to be caused by it, and is often largely the result of a faulty immune system, weakened by Candida.

41

NOTE

Only one thing needs correcting in Sue's story. The stopping of yeast-based foods is not because this 'feeds the yeast' but rather because the system of the person thus affected will usually have become sensitized to yeasts, and eating foods based on yeast, or containing moulds, will further irritate and aggravate this situation.

Understanding Candida

It is clear that the ramifications of Candida infection are not yet fully understood, and that much clarification and research remains to be done. In the mean time, since it is not difficult to identify reasons to suspect its possible involvement, it seems reasonable that a Candida control programme should be adopted in cases where a combination of both a history and symptoms exist, where there is a pattern of ill health similar to any of those touched on above, whatever previous diagnosis has been made.

The treatment is, after all, harmless and indeed health-promoting.

All in the Mind?

Other conditions which are sometimes confused with Candida involvement are frequently labelled as psychosomatic. This can be a way for doctors to avoid having to say that they cannot find the cause. Calling conditions such as this 'functional' or 'psychosomatic' may, if repeated, result in patients beginning to believe that they really are not quite balanced. The terms 'neurotic' and 'nervous' are often ascribed to such individuals, with devastating effects on morale and self-esteem. The yeast or fungal cause may remain unsuspected, or, if noted as part of the problem (if thrush is a part of the 'psychosomatic' symptom picture, for example), be simply ignored as a minor piece of the puzzle, unworthy of therapeutic effort.

In Chronic Fatigue Syndrome/ME this sort of labelling has led to extreme anger which has been focused into patient self-help efforts and the emergence of insistent demands for a more scientific examination of their condition. Organizations such as Action for ME and Chronic Fatigue, which has done so much in the UK for ME to be taken seriously, were in fact the result of the frustration of people such as Sue Finlay at being told that their health problems were psychologically based.

There is reason to believe that Candida infection is a rampant problem in modern society. It has been let loose by the use of drugs, used in good faith to help in other directions, as well as by a dietary pattern which is ideal for the sustenance of the yeast, rather than the host. The number and variety of possible consequences is mind-boggling and deserves the attention of every individual involved in the healing professions.

The alertness of one man, Dr Truss, has brought about the current increase in awareness of the significance of Candida. He may not be totally right in his concept, but the results he has so far obtained in thousands of cases bearing a range of symptoms such as those already discussed simply by paying attention to the yeast component of the problem are proof of the validity of this method of treatment.

There is no area of health more amenable to self-assessment and self-help, and the information which will be provided in subsequent chapters should enable improvement in most cases in which Candida is the main culprit, or where it is a part of the cause of symptoms.

The questionnaire on the following pages will give you the chance to assess the possibility of Candida being a major part of your current health picture. It is possible for most of the symptoms described to be the result of causes other than

Candida. If, however, you have more than one of the indications on List 2, as well as some of the lesser symptoms listed at the end of the questionnaire, then the possibility increases to a probability, especially if you can identify a possible causative link with at least one of the factors in List 1.

Candida Albicans Checklist

Completing this questionnaire will give you clues as to whether Candida is an active agent in your current health spectrum. It is not possible to make a diagnosis by these means alone, but a strong indication, as evidenced by positive answers in all sections of the questionnaire, is possible and can be used to assist you in deciding whether to undertake a Candida control programme.

List 1: History of Drug Usage, etc.

1 Have you ever taken a course of antibiotics for an infectious condition which lasted for either eight weeks or longer, or for short periods four or more times in one year? ❏
2 Have you ever taken a course of antibiotics for the treatment of acne for a month or more continuously? ❏
3 Have you ever had a course of steroid treatment such as prednisone, cortisone or ACTH? ❏
4 Have you ever taken contraceptive medication for a year or more? ❏
5 Have you ever been treated with immuno-suppressant drugs? ❏
6 Have you been pregnant more than once? ❏

TOTAL:

List 2: Major Symptom History (Candida Implicated)

 1 Have you in the past had recurrent or persistent cystitis, vaginitis or prostatitis? ❑

 2 Have you a history of endometriosis? ❑

 3 Have you had thrush (oral or vaginal) more than once? ❑

 4 Have you ever had athlete's foot or a fungal infection of the nails or skin? ❑

 5 Are you severely affected by exposure to chemical fumes, perfumes, tobacco smoke, etc.? Or are your symptoms worse after taking yeasty or sugary foods or drinks? ❑

 6 Do you suffer from a variety of allergies? ❑

 7 Do you commonly suffer from abdominal distension, 'bloating', diarrhoea or constipation? ❑

 8 Do you suffer from premenstrual syndrome (fluid retention, irritability, etc.)? ❑

 9 Do you suffer from depression, fatigue, lethargy, poor memory, feelings of 'unreality'? ❑

10 Do you crave sweet foods, bread or alcohol? ❑

11 Do you suffer from unaccountable muscle aches, tingling, numbness or burning? ❑

12 Do you suffer from unaccountable aches and swelling in joints? ❑

13 Do you have vaginal discharge or irritation, or menstrual cramp or pain? ❑

14 Do you have erratic vision or spots before the eyes? ❑

15 Do you suffer from impotence or lack of sexual desire? ❑

TOTAL:

If you have answered Yes to one or more questions in the first section, and to two or more in the second section, as well as some of the following being present, then Candida is probably involved in causing your symptoms:

- symptoms usually worse on damp days
- persistent drowsiness
- lack of co-ordination
- headaches
- mood swings
- loss of balance
- rashes
- mucus in stools
- belching and 'wind'
- bad breath
- dry mouth
- post-nasal drip
- nasal itch and/or congestion
- nervous irritability
- tightness in chest
- dry mouth or throat
- ear sensitivity or fluid in ears
- heartburn and indigestion.

Life-threatening Implications of Candida

We have looked at some of the common, sometimes serious – sometimes merely nuisance – results of Candida overgrowth. We should take note, though, that life itself may be threatened by specific combinations of infection which can result when our immune function is low and Candida is active. Before we discuss research evidence of a terrible symbiosis between *Staphylococcus aureus* and Candida albicans (both of which, incidentally, can be controlled naturally by friendly bacteria such as acidophilus), we should briefly examine some of the known disease states which *Staphylococcus aureus* is known to produce.

Toxic Shock Syndrome (TSS)

This is typically found in young women (95 per cent of cases). Those affected by TSS begin to notice symptoms on about the fifth day of their period (tampons are usually being used). Symptoms include a widespread rash, fever, watery diarrhoea, vomiting, sore throat, headaches and aching muscles. The skin may begin to peel off, kidney failure may ensue and both respiratory and cardiac complications are common. One or two out of every ten people affected by TSS die.

The cause is rampant infestation with *Staphylococcus aureus*, with the symptoms being largely the result of toxins which this bacteria produces.

Scalded Skin Syndrome (SSS)

This condition affects infants, young children and immune-suppressed adults, and usually follows a spread of *Staphylococcus aureus* from a primary infection somewhere else in the body such as conjunctivitis. SSS is characterized by fever and profound weakness and a bright red, very tender, skin rash involving large blisters which slough off in sheets of skin, leaving large areas of the body without skin at all. Even normal-looking skin shears away with light pressure. Complications occur relating to the body's temperature control and fluid balance mechanisms being disrupted in this way. As with TSS, this is caused by a toxin secreted by the Staphylococcus bacteria.

Between 80 and 90 per cent of *Staphylococcus aureus* infections which are found in hospital settings are 'super infections', resistant to antibiotics. Other conditions associated with *Staphylococcus aureus* include gastroenteritis, bone and joint infections (osteomyelitis) and septic arthritis, pneumonia, meningitis, inflammatory heart disease, etc.

The Candida Connection with TSS and SSS

In a series of experiments Dr Eunice Carlson of the University of Michigan established that when there was a combined infection of *Staphylococcus aureus* (or *Streptococcus faecalis* or *Serratia marcescens*) and Candida albicans there was an enormous potentiation of the infection caused by the bacteria. She tells us, 'Although these studies show that Candida has a strong amplifying effect on the virulence of other organisms (*Staphylococcus aureus, Streptococcus faecalis*) how this is achieved is a mystery.'[6]

She continues:

One possibility is that the candidal infection progress causes physical damage to the organ walls which makes them 'leaky' allowing other microbes or chemicals (perhaps toxins), or both, to penetrate more easily: it is also possible that Candida directly stimulates the growth of Staphylococcus aureus.

It is not difficult to understand one of Dr Carlson's explanations, since we already know of Candida's ability to make tissues 'leaky', as in the digestive tract, when it changes from its yeast form to its aggressive fungal stage.

Dr Carlson looks at the almost inexplicable fact that Candida is seldom automatically dealt with by doctors, and gives the example of Candida infection related to denture wearing.

This is now believed to be very common and to occur in 60 per cent of all denture wearers. Biopsies of inflamed areas however consistently fail to demonstrate tissue invasion (with Candida). We can speculate that an equivalent infection of the small intestine would be virtually undetectable.

So because Candida's presence is not obvious it is ignored!

One of the most important messages this book can give is that we have to assume Candida's active presence on the basis of the person's symptoms and history, not on expensive, time-consuming scientific tests, which are commonly inconclusive.

Dr Carlson continues,

Physicians have reported therapeutic cures for a variety of diverse disease conditions using anti-candidal drugs. It now appears possible that this fungus may play a key role in many disease conditions, not by its own toxic or invasive growth, but rather by enhancing secondary infection.

The methods outlined in the following chapters are suitable for preventing the sort of ailments which Candida produces on its own, and also for the disasters which are possible (TSS and SSS, for example) when other infections occur alongside it.

Candida and Chronic Disease

As we have seen earlier in this chapter, Dr Truss has reported on apparent multiple sclerosis and schizophrenia patients recovering their health when Candida was tackled. Other researchers have pointed to additional connections between yeast overgrowth and a variety of serious health problems.

British researcher Sheridan Stock has identified a number of ways in which Candida overgrowth can contribute towards a weakening of adrenal gland function (this is the gland which produces adrenalin, the 'energy' hormone) as well as thyroid function.[7]

He states 'The functioning of the thyroid gland is one of the first activities interfered with by Candida and it has been observed that 90 per cent of Candida victims have low thyroid function.'[8]

Underactivity of adrenal and/or thyroid glands can lead to inadequate hormonal secretions (or an inability of the hormones to act normally) and produces symptoms which could include extreme fatigue, depression, weight gain, dry skin and sensitivity to cold.

Stock has also linked Candida activity to many children with learning disabilities and hyperactivity. He reports:

> *Mothers of hyperactive children often give a history of candidal vaginitis, particularly during pregnancy, and the children have often been exposed to antibiotics early in life. A low income is frequently part of the picture and leads to poor nutrition and a high-sugar diet.*

Almost all people with HIV/AIDS or other immune-compromised conditions have Candida infections. Eileen Stretch, a Canadian physician, reports that unexplained vaginal candidiasis which resists treatment is often the only sign of underlying immune deficiency."

NOTE
This does not mean that everyone with chronic Candida problems is severely immune deficient, but that everyone who is severely immune deficient is likely to have Candida overgrowth as a major part of their symptom picture.

In the UK, cancer expert Dr Nadia Coates has stated that she does not believe that cancer develops unless there is a yeast overgrowth in the small intestines which causes damage which then allows absorption through its mucous membranes of toxic wastes.[10]

A wide range of other chronic conditions, including some forms of arthritis, incapacitating migraines, prostatitis, endometriosis, disabling cystitis, extreme chronic fatigue and widespread allergic symptoms can all be caused by Candida activity.

Once again it is necessary to clarify this by saying that these conditions may also be the result of other causes, but that

Candida is frequently a major factor.

The questionnaire listed earlier can give you strong indications as to whether or not yeast is likely to be a factor in any symptoms you are suffering. The next chapters will guide you towards controlling this.

Chapter 5

CONTROLLING CANDIDA NATURALLY

– SUPPLEMENTS AND HERBAL EXTRACTS

If after reading the information in the past four chapters, and answering the questionnaire, it seems to you that Candida is a likely suspect as a cause of your condition, then it is necessary to prove this by means of adopting an anti-Candida programme. If this succeeds in making a major impact upon your health, by virtue of its controlling Candida and improving your symptom picture, then you will have proved your assumption to be correct. Dr W. M. Crook calls this 'a therapeutic trial'.[1] It is really the only way of being absolutely sure, since there is as yet no way of discovering whether Candida is involved by any laboratory tests.

This is a stumbling block for many people. They want 'cast-iron proof' that Candida is the culprit. None the less all we can do is look at the picture that is currently present in your particular condition and add to this a review of your past history. If that looks like a 'Candida picture', then there really is no other choice, apart from going on as you are, than to introduce anti-Candida measures.

If a culture were made of your fluid discharges, tissues or excreta, it would inevitably display Candida's presence somewhere in your body. This would not prove or disprove anything, as far as your symptoms are concerned, since a positive test result could also be obtained from almost every adult in the land, with and without symptoms.

Only by looking at the known and suspected pattern of symptom production that has been built up around Candida's activity can we guess its active presence (as opposed to its benign presence if your immune system and intestinal flora are keeping it under control). The only real proof is in the treatment results. If you are better after controlling Candida, then you will know that what you assumed was accurate and that your programme was the correct one. The very least that you will achieve is that you will have reformed your dietary pattern, and will have swallowed some harmless vitamins and other supplements, as well as building up your immune system's ability to combat its adversaries.

It would be quite reasonable to question whether it is really necessary to attack Candida which may be obviously active in a local region (oral or vaginal thrush for example) by an approach which is aimed at the intestinal tract as well. Fortunately there is now clear evidence that this is the right way to tackle the problem.

Researchers writing in the *American Journal of Obstetrics and Gynecology* detailed their findings in which they treated women with serious vulvo-vaginal candidiasis. These people were also assessed for intestinal Candida activity, and in all 258 women involved this was shown to be evident. The patients were divided into two groups, one of which received antifungal medication both by mouth (for the intestines) and vaginally. The other group had antifungal medication locally for the vagina but took a dummy tablet (placebo). The medication was used for just one week and the women were reassessed after one week, three weeks and seven weeks.

The results showed that 88 per cent of those receiving both the digestive tract and local antifungal approach were clear of

Candida overgrowth, as against 75 per cent of those who had intravaginal therapy alone. While this shows significant, although not massive, benefits when both the local (vaginal) and the intestinal Candida are treated simultaneously, there is an even more important result when both are attacked: a reduction in recurrence, which is far higher among women not also aggressively treated for digestive yeast overgrowth.

What this means is that if you treat local thrush and/or yeast-induced vaginitis locally, without treating the overgrowth in the intestinal tract, you will probably improve but there will be an equal probability of a rapid recurrence. If the intestinal overgrowth is treated, however, recurrence becomes far less likely.

Controlling Candida falls into three different segments. First there are a number of nutrient and probiotic supplements which help to control Candida, largely by encouraging healthy bowel flora and supporting immune function. Secondly there are a number of plant-based antifungal medications, many of which should be prescribed only by a health professional.

These two strands of the anti-Candida programme will be described in this chapter, along with some specialized advice for local (oral, vaginal, for example) yeast problems.

Finally, but absolutely vitally, in the next chapter a pattern of eating will be described which is designed to 'starve' yeast of its favourite foods, depriving Candida of its growth potential. In that chapter suggestions will also be given regarding avoidance of foods which might provoke allergic-type reactions in those who have become yeast-sensitive.

In this chapter we will also review some tactics which may be necessary if the digestive tract has become inflamed or irritated by the activity of Candida.

Repopulation of Friendly Bacteria – Probiotics[3]

When antibiotics are used they destroy a number of 'friendly' bacteria which inhabit our digestive tract, and which, as well as providing other valuable symbiotic (mutually beneficial) contributions to the body's economy, also act as a controlling element in stopping Candida from spreading.

In the average bowel there exist huge colonies of micro-organisms which in total weight come to between 3 and 5 lb and in number exceed the total number of cells in your body. These are not all helpful or friendly, however, and in order to repopulate the bowel with helpful residents such as acidophilus and bifidobacteria, large quantities of the friendly varieties need to be supplemented. When these recolonize, intruders such as Candida are pushed back and often eliminated from the area.

Dr Khem Shehani, one of the world's leading researchers into probiotics (therapeutic use of friendly bacteria) and their medicinal properties, is quite clear on the usefulness of the *lactobacilli* against yeast infections. 'Continuing research has revealed that supplementing the diet with friendly bacteria, like acidophilus and other compatible organisms such as *Bifidobacteria bifidum* ... should help in curing candidiasis.'[4]

This viewpoint is confirmed by Japanese research (in 1984) which examined the degree of overgrowth of Candida as ascertained by the levels found in the faeces of patients with leukaemia who were receiving drug therapy. The Candida counts were very high indeed, before treatment with bifidobacteria (this is the friendly bacteria which inhabits the large intestine, unlike acidophilus which lives mainly in the small intestine). Bifidobacteria supplementation had the effect of reducing the levels of Candida in the faeces of some patients from a high of 10,000,000 per gram to a mere 10,000 per gram, after treatment.

The effectiveness of bifidobacteria in achieving this was seen in all 16 patients treated, whereas 11 'control' patients not receiving bifidobacteria supplementation showed no change at all in their Candida levels.

Many researchers report that *Lactobacillus acidophilus* (and bifidobacteria) seems actually to manufacture substances which retard the growth of Candida, and this is borne out when *Lactobacillus acidophilus* is added to culture dishes in which Candida is growing, where an ability is seen to slow and even stop its growth.

An additional bonus is received when bifidobacteria are supplemented against Candida, as this has a uniquely powerful ability to enhance detoxification via the liver, as well as its extremely useful detoxifying role in the intestinal tract itself.

For these many reasons I can only echo the words of leading American nutrition expert Dr Jeffrey Bland, when he states:[3]

> *We have been very excited about an alternative therapy for the management of Candida infection, which avoids the use of anti-yeast medication (nystatin, etc.). It is well recognized that a disturbed flora of the GI [gastro-intestinal] tract can establish a proper environment for yeast proliferation. By reinoculating (supplementation of) the bowel with the proper symbiotic acid producing bacteria* (Lactobacillus acidophilus *and bifidobacteria) there is a reduction in the compatibility of the intestinal environment for the yeast proliferation. We have recently used an oral supplement of* Lactobacillus acidophilus... *this has been extremely successful in reducing Candida albicans in the intestinal tract. The* Lactobacillus acidophilus *is given as a dry culture.*

This approach of using friendly bacteria to repopulate the digestive tract will be seen to play a major part in the strategy which I outline below. This is suitable for anyone with active Candida overgrowth.

These (*Lactobacillus acidophilus* and bifidobacteria) are therefore the first of the anti-Candida supplements you should introduce, together with live cultured yogurt and/or sour milk with meals (as long as you are not allergic to dairy products).

Two of the major probiotic 'bacterial friends' which we have are *Lactobacillus acidophilus* and *Bifidus*. If sufficient of these bacteria can be encouraged to re-establish residence, in the small and large intestines respectively, this will help to control yeast which may have crowded into the vacant space left when antibiotics (or other factors such as an imbalanced high-sugar/high-fat diet) destroyed or weakened acidophilus and bifidus colonies.

An additional boost to the efficient function of these friendly bacteria is a non-resident organism, *Lactobacillus bulgaricus*, one of the yogurt-making (together with *Thermophilus*) bacteria.

Bacterial cultures which are meant for supplementation are available in a number of forms, as powders or in capsules. Cultured milk products containing acidophilus and bifidus organisms can also play a part in the anti-Candida programme, although the numbers present in such products are relatively low compared with the high-potency powders and capsules currently available.

Essential Probiotic Knowledge[6]

When acidophilus or bifidobacteria are supplemented it is vital to ensure that the product you are taking contains not less than 1 billion viable, active (potential colony-forming) organisms per gram. This almost always means that the product will need to be kept refrigerated once it has been opened, and cool at all times. The potency (number of organisms per gram) needs to be guaranteed at the time of purchase – not at the time of manufacture.

When taking these two organisms therapeutically – as in an

anti-Candida programme – they should be taken in equal quantities, in water. The amount taken will vary with the condition but is usually in the range of 5 to 10 grams daily of each, in divided doses between meals, for a week or more, followed by half that quantity for the duration of the programme, which usually runs for three to six months, depending on progress.

A lesser 'maintenance' dose is commonly suggested for long-term use.

A rough guide is that a teaspoonful of powdered probiotic culture is equal to about 2 grams, which – depending on potency – equals around 2 to 3 billion organisms of each type with each teaspoonful.

Powders are usually suggested to be taken two to three times daily between meals, whereas encapsulated products are commonly suggested to be taken with meals.

A supplement of *Lactobacillus bulgaricus* is also often suggested, in powder form, in a dosage of around a teaspoonful of pow-dered culture with each meal as an immune-enhancing strategy as well as to improve the colonizing ability of acidophilus and bifidus.

Children under the age of seven should be supplemented with *Bifidobacteria infantis* and *not* the adult version, and not with acidophilus unless there has been a recent infection or use of antibiotics, in which case they should be supplemented with both in a ratio of 50:50.

A 35-kg (77-lb/5½-st) child should take half the adult quantity of probiotic organisms; a 20-kg (44-lb/3-st) child, or less, a quarter of the adult dose.

Precautions when supplementing with Probiotics:

1   It is suggested that probiotic products which contain additional organisms other than acidophilus, bifidobacteria or bulgaricus, such as *Streptococcus faecium* and *Lactobacillus casei*, for example, should be avoided. The reason for these

being included in mixtures of 'somethingdophilus' is usually a commercial one; there are few dangers – only a loss of quality and a waste of money.

2   Ensure that the container in which the organisms are purchased is of dark glass, and that there is a guarantee of potency up to an expiry date on the label, and that refrigeration is recommended.

3   Avoid liquid probiotic products – stick with powders (best) or capsules. Avoid tablets, as the process of manufacture destroys much of the potential of the organisms to colonize.

4   If possible, ensure (ask the retailer or manufacturer) that the product was not centrifuged when the organisms where separated from the supernatant (the 'soup' in which they are grown), as this is a damaging process for them and reduces their colonizing potential.

5   Try to obtain specific strains of the organisms, for example LB-51, a super-efficient strain of *L. bulgaricus*, and DDS-1, which is a well-documented super-strain of acidophilus.

6   If you are dairy sensitive make sure that the culture was not grown on a dairy base. Many other options are available from the better manufacturers.

7   Wherever possible obtain each organism in a separate container, as they are not compatible with each other when kept together even if freeze-dried. An exception to this is found in the British product BioAcidophilus (BioCare product) which contains both acidophilus and bifidobacteria, kept apart by a special process of micro-encapsulation.

8 Follow the manufacturer's advice regarding when the product should be taken.

9 Do not be confused by claims that particular products are 'human strains' or 'human compatible'. All high-quality probiotic products are suitable for human use, and in the UK this includes products manufactured by Natren, BioCare, Blackmore, Lamberts, Solgar, NF Formulas, Higher Nature, Quest and others. If you ask the questions which this list suggests you will obtain products of a quality appropriate for an anti-Candida programme.

10 Many practitioners suggest waiting for a week or two after commencing an anti-Candida programme before starting supplementation with probiotics. I prefer to start with them immediately as they actually enhance detoxification of the waste products of yeast which is dying off, and the sooner recolonization can start the better. If the gut wall has become inflamed due to Candida activity recolonization may be slower than is ideal, however there are strategies which are suggested below to assist in this.

The products which I normally recommend, based on their use by thousands of patients for over 15 years, are those manufactured by Natren, who usually recommend that their products should be taken away from meal times (an hour before, ideally), and BioCare products which are usually suggested to be taken with meals. This does not mean that there is no value in other products, only that these are the ones I prefer.

Biotin

Another major nutrient employed against Candida activity which is taken with probiotic supplements is the B-vitamin biotin.

Research in Japan has indicated a fascinating way in which Candida can be deterred from altering from its relatively harmless yeast form into its invasive and dangerously mycelial form.[7]

This alteration of form is found to occur more rapidly in a medium in which there is a relative biotin deficiency. Biotin, which has also been called vitamin H, produces a number of skin conditions when known deficiency occurs in humans. These include a dermatitis which is characterized by a greyish, dry, flaky appearance. This is accompanied by a lack of appetite, nausea, lassitude and muscular pains. It is interesting that all of these symptoms are common when Candida is proliferating, and it is worth questioning whether the supposed symptoms of biotin deficiency are not at least in part the result of Candida activity brought about by that deficiency.

Egg-white contains a substance called avidin, which is capable of combining with biotin, thus neutralizing its usefulness in the body. For this reason raw egg should not be included in the anti-Candida diet (avidin is destroyed by cooking).

Biotin should be taken as a supplement, three times daily, in doses of between 350 and 500 mcg in association with acidophilus (i.e. between meals).

Antifungal Strategies

Aloe Vera Juice

The juice of the desert plant Aloe vera is a powerful antifungal agent.

The amazing healing qualities of Aloe vera have been known since Phoenician times. In recent years attention has been drawn to its usefulness in a range of digestive conditions. Professor Jeffrey Bland has demonstrated that the activity of the fresh juice on Candida can be very helpful to sufferers. He writes:

> *In a study of ten subjects, six had markedly altered stool cultures in microbiological assays. Four of these had indications of yeast overgrowth in their stools, before taking Aloe vera, and had reduction in yeast abundance after Aloe vera supplementation. Aloe vera has an antifungal action as well as improving overall bowel flora condition and improving the local acidity balance.[8]*

As Bland says, 'It promotes a favourable balance of gastro-intestinal symbiotic bacteria.'

It has a similar effect on bacterial and fungal infection on the skin, and can be applied to such conditions locally.

One or two teaspoonful of Aloe vera juice in water should be taken twice daily by anyone with Candida problems. (*Note:* Once opened, Aloe vera juice should be kept refrigerated. The optimum shelf-life thereafter is about one month.)

Garlic (allicin)

Garlic has been the subject of research world-wide. Russian scientists have proved the reality of its long-reputed antibacterial quality by introducing garlic extract into colonies of bacteria, which ceased to function within minutes. Fresh garlic juice was employed in these tests. Reports in Western medical and scientific journals confirm such claims,[9] in this case against *Salmonella typhimurium* and *Escherichia coli*, two extremely active micro-organisms. Garlic is also active against yeast and fungi. This was confirmed in recent reports showing it to be more active against human ringworm (a fungal infection) than currently used drugs.[10]

The *Book of Garlic* quotes researchers as stating, 'garlic in the form of juice is a very potent anti-microbial agent, both to bacteria, and Pathogenic yeasts. We can thus suppose at least staphylococcal and fungal skin and alimentary tract disease can be effectively cured by the juice of garlic.'[11]

Research at the University of Indiana suggests that the value of garlic against fungal infections is very great. 'An aqueous extract of garlic bulbs inhibits growth of many aspects of zoopathogenic fungi,' the first report stated.[12]

The second concluded that Allicin, the active sulphur-rich compound in garlic, 'may provide the model system for chemotherapy of Candida albicans infections'.[13]

The aesthetic aspect of garlic's employment is of course a factor to consider. While there are many who can happily eat whole cloves of garlic, there are others who find the taste and odour unpleasant. The recent development of a completely odourless garlic is a boon to such as these. (*See Further Information for suppliers.*)

Part of your anti-Candida campaign should include the daily intake of either fresh garlic or deodorized garlic in capsule form. The former is preferred; the latter is an acceptable compromise. Take two to three garlic capsules, morning and evening, after meals, or eat as much raw garlic as you can learn to enjoy. Slice it finely on cooked vegetables, or crush it onto salads, or simply eat it, clove by clove, with fish or poultry, as many Greeks do.

Olive Oil (oleic acid)

A further aid in the prevention of the transformation of Candida to its mycelial form is the use of olive oil.[14]

This contains a substance called oleic acid, which acts upon the yeast in a similar way to biotin. The recommended amount of olive oil is six teaspoonsful daily, divided into three doses. This can be included in the meal or taken before or after, as desired.

Anti-Candida Herbs

Tea Tree Oil (Maleluca alternofolia)

An extract of this Australian plant has powerful antifungal properties. Douching daily with a 1 per cent solution in water (or once weekly soaking a tampon which is then inserted vaginally for no more than 24 hours) can be very useful for vaginitis or cervicitis. This approach is useful whether the cause is Candida or trichomoniasis. Tea tree oil can also be used as a gargle or mouthwash (one drop in a tumbler of water) for oral thrush, and directly onto the skin when in an ointment base (it is somewhat irritating to the skin if used neat as an oil). Another use is as a pessary for vaginal thrush.

Chamomile (Matricaria chamomilla)

Chamomile contains antifungal substances in its oily extracts. Used as a tea or topical application it has soothing qualities, as has taheebo (Pau D'Arco – *see page 67*), which is derived from the South American plant *Tabebuia avellanedae* which has strong anti-Candida (and anti-tumour) effects.

The most powerful anti-Candida herbs contain berberine, such as *Berberis vulgaris* (barberry), *Hydrastis canadensis* (golden-seal) and *Berberis aquifolium* (Oregon grape). Berberine's action against Candida prevents overgrowth after antibiotic use, and also helps repopulate the gut with friendly bacteria. Berberine is an anti-diarrhoea agent when chronic bowel infection is involved and also has immune system-enhancing capabilities as it destroys bacteria, yeasts, viruses and cancer cells ... quite a catalogue of benefits.

Another similar effect is found with use of the herb *Echinacea angustifolia* (purple coneflower), which has been used for centuries in Native American medicine. It is a powerful antiviral and antifungal agent and an immune system enhancer. An excellent American product (EHB – manufactured by NF Formulas) combines echinacea, hydrastis and berberine together with immune-enhancing nutrients such as zinc and vitamin C.

Dosage suggestions

1 to 3 EHB capsules daily or

1 to 2 grams of dried bark or root of *Berberis vulgaris* or *Hydrastis canadensis* (powdered or as a tea) three times daily

or

1 to 1½ teaspoons (4 to 6 ml) of tincture of either of these plants (diluted 1:5), three times daily, or

¼ to ½ a teaspoon of fluid extract of either of these plants, three times daily.

Anti-parasitic Herbs and Plant Extracts

A new development has been the use of extracts of citrus (usually grapefruit) seeds as a safe, natural anti-Candida and antiparasitic agent. This extract is not absorbed into the system or tissues and is non-toxic. It can take several months of supplementation to eliminate common parasites such as *Giardia lamblia* which are frequently found in association with Candida overgrowth.

Additional anti-parasitic herbal assistance is found in the use of berberine (as discussed above) and also *Artemisia annua*, a traditional Chinese herb which is commonly combined with grapefruit seed extract as an antifungal and antiparasitic medicine. This should not be confused with *Artemisia absinthum*, a traditional European herb which can be toxic and the use of which is illegal in some countries.

A number of safe antiparasitic herbal combinations are available at health food stores. Most are effective against both yeasts and parasites, for example BioCare's Eradicidin Forte which contains berberine, Artemisia and grapefruit seed extract.

Caprylic Acid

The antifungal activity of certain fatty acids has been demonstrated by investigators such as Neuhauser,[13] who has shown dilute (0.01) caprylic acid (coconut extract) to destroy Candida effectively. He has successfully treated patients with severe intestinal Candida by using caprylic acid in a form which allows a timed release as it passes through the bowel. If not in such a form the caprylic acid is ineffective, being absorbed in the upper intestinal region. Caprylic acid mimics the fatty acids produced by normal bowel flora, which are a major factor in the body's control over Candida. Caprylic acid is now widely available in the UK (*see Further Information for details*).

The formulation of caprylic acid most widely used in the UK, and which is recommended for the programme outlined in this book, is Mycopryl (BioCare), which is produced in various strengths for use in severe and mild conditions as well as for children and in maintenance settings (*see page 117*).

Dosage (to accompany dietary antifungal strategies)

If Candida is mild it is suggested that you take Mycopryl 400, one capsule with each meal, for the first two months; then reduce to Mycopryl 250 with each meal for a further two months.

If Candida is severe take Mycopryl 680 for the first two months, then reduce to Mycopryl 400 for the next two months.

Children should take Mycopryl 250 as part of a comprehensive anti-yeast programme.

If yeast 'die-off' (*see notes later in this chapter*) is producing a strong reaction, then the dose of Mycopryl should be reduced for a few days (take half the prescribed amount, for example) until detoxification has cleared the debris which is causing the symptoms.

Supplementation with zinc and molybdenum has been found to assist in the detoxification process.

Caprylic acid is recommended in preference to the commonly employed antifungal medical drugs such as nystatin (which is discussed below), because the latter is itself yeast-based and research at the Washington University School of Medicine shows that ultimately, after a period of treatment, when nystatin is stopped it often results in even more colonies of yeast developing than were present before its use. Caprylic acid has no such rebound effect when its use ceases after Candida is controlled (we never actually get rid of the yeast, remember, but only try to get it back under control).

Undecylenic Acid (Castor-bean Extract)

A fatty acid, undecylenic acid (which is also found naturally in our sweat) is derived from the castor bean has been found by some researchers to be at least as effective an antifungal as caprylic acid, and under ideal conditions more effective. This is a major ingredient of the formulation 'Phytostatin', which also contains caprylic acid, grapefruit seed extract and extract of Pau D'Arco (NF Formulas). These fatty acids are delivered to the appropriate part of the digestive tract by means of time-release capsules, so ensuring that they are not absorbed too high up in the tract.

Tannate Plant Extracts

Plant extracts called tannates (such as tannin in tea) are powerful antifungal agents. When taken orally (as 'Tanalbit') they destroy yeasts selectively, including their spores, without harming the natural flora of the body. There are also formulations for use in the mouth when Candida is locally active ('Tanoral') and for intravaginal use when thrush is evident ('Tanafem').

An advantage of using tannates is that they act only in the digestive tract, not being absorbed at all, unlike fatty acids which may be absorbed unless delivered in suitable time-release capsules.

These tannates, manufactured in the USA by NF Formulas, are also useful in detoxifying heavy metals from the body, and are therefore suitable for use when mercury toxicity, for example, is a factor in immune suppression, as described in Chapter 2.

Up to six (usually three) capsules of 600 mg each are suggested with each meal for at least two and ideally up to eight weeks for chronic candidiasis.

CAUTION
None of the herbal formulations such as echinacea or the tannates should be used by pregnant women.

Medical Antifungal Strategies

Nystatin
The orthodox medical treatment of fungal infection, such as Candida, by drug methods involves the use of antifungal antibiotics such as nystatin. This substance is active against a wide range of yeasts and yeast-like fungi, including Candida. This drug comes in a variety of forms: as a liquid, for use in the mouth; as tablets, for use in treating Candida in the intestinal tract; as suppositories, for use in the vagina; and as creams, ointments and powders, for the treatment of surface areas, nails, etc. Some of the reasons for urging caution in long-term use of nystatin have been given in earlier chapters. Discussion of it in this section, which deals with antifungal strategies, is for information only and is not meant as a recommendation. Nystatin is suggested as a safe and helpful drug by authorities such as William Crook MD, whose book *The Yeast Connection* has done so much to encourage

awareness of the damage candidiasis can cause. The fact is that, despite assurances from Crook and other experts that nystatin only acts inside the digestive tract, it seems likely that where the gut wall has been damaged by yeast some of the drug may enter the bloodstream with unpredictable results.

Activist author Gill Jacobs points out another possibility in her excellent book *Candida Albicans – a user's guide to treatment and recovery*. She observes that nystatin is a polyene antibiotic and that such substances have been found actually to boost the numbers of yeast cells which can actively colonize in our tissues.[16]

Other Antifungal Drugs

There are a number of other commonly used antifungal drugs which have various drawbacks when compared with the safer natural substances which are discussed in this book.

Diflucan (flucanazole)
This expensive drug has been found to require lengthy use to have any noticeable effect.

Amphotericin B
Known as fungalin, this has similarities with nystatin. It has been banned in the USA. It is known to be toxic when used intravenously, and this must raise doubts as to safety because of the possibility of absorption through a damaged gut wall.

Nizoral (ketonazole)
Nizoral causes damage to the liver as a result of its easy access to the bloodstream from the intestinal tract.

In medical settings none of these drugs is usually used with a comprehensive antifungal dietary and supplement approach which would encourage a healthier digestive tract and immune system.

None of them is necessary at all, since the methods which are outlined in this and later chapters are safer and of proven efficacy.

Nystatin is lethal to yeast cells on contact. Getting them into contact with the drug is not always easy, especially if the area involved is deep in the bowel. The nystatin, passing through, will kill surface yeasts, but any that are embedded deeper into the wall of the intestine will remain untouched. There is poor absorption of nystatin, so little reaches the bloodstream.

There is a general consensus that nystatin is well tolerated and causes few side-effects.[17] The major reason for not opting for its use is that it deals only with the short-term situation and that yeast can become tolerant of it. If a condition such as Candida has become so widespread as to cause a problem, then it is vital that the immune system and bowel flora, which should be controlling the situation, are revitalized. Reliance on nystatin will leave the immune system in the same state, except that there will, over a period of time, be fewer yeast byproducts entering the bloodstream to challenge the immune system. This, it is thought (Truss, Crook, etc.), allows the immune system to revive gradually. There is certainly no objection to nystatin being employed if the condition is severe enough to warrant it, but this should only be done in combination with the sort of programme outlined in this book. Otherwise there will be only short-term gains and the condition will recur. It is important to realize that nystatin is itself derived from a mould source and can cause allergic symptoms in sensitive individuals. Some patients become dependent on nystatin and find it difficult to be weaned off it. One of the more distressing factors relating to long-term use of nystatin is the likelihood of a 'rebound' of yeast activity when it is stopped.

The dosage of nystatin (available in UK as 'Nystan') is usually around 2 million units daily (4 tablets of 500,000 units each), but double this dosage is relatively safe. Side-effects are limited to nausea, vomiting and diarrhoea, which occur only with very high doses (over 4 million units daily).

The major recommendations given in this book regarding the control of Candida by *natural* rather than drug methods are effective in the majority of cases. Taking nystatin does not necessarily shorten the process of control, and indeed may result in the individual relying on the drug and thus allowing the supporting anti-Candida programme to lapse.

By relying on the supplementation programme outlined in this chapter together with the dietary guidelines in the next chapter, it is possible not only to control Candida but to improve your general well-being dramatically. This is something no drug can achieve, however few side-effects it produces.

Immune-System
Enhancement by Supplementation

In order to strengthen the immune system it is suggested that a number of essential nutrients be included in the programme. Not all of these may be needed in each case, and it is only by taking expert advice that your particular needs can be assessed.

The importance of vitamin C cannot be over-emphasized. T-cells, which form a major part of our defence system, contain high levels of vitamin C. It has been noted that the lower the vitamin C content of these vital cells the less efficient is their performance in defending the body against intruding organisms or materials, including yeast.[18]

Any stress, whether originating in the emotions or caused by the presence of toxic pollution, infection, or other factors, places demands upon the vitamin C levels in the body. This is a water-soluble vitamin and the body has no stores of it, so a constant supply is needed. Research has shown a fascinating adaptation which takes place when requirements increase because of stress or infection.

Under normal conditions, if a person takes more vitamin C than he or she actually requires, the person is likely to develop a degree of diarrhoea. This is well known and is a way of assessing just how much vitamin C you need. If someone takes 5 g daily, with no diarrhoea resulting, then he or she can be assumed to need that amount, at that time. If under normal conditions, however, someone develops diarrhoea after ingesting only 2 g daily, it can be shown that should circumstances alter and the need for vitamin C increase (owing to infection, stress, etc.) then that same person could increase vitamin C intake even by many times 2 g daily without any bowel symptoms at all. Dr Robert Cathcart has shown that if necessary the intake of vitamin C can be as high as 100 g a day (never try this without supervision), with no bowel sensitivity apparent.[19]

When the crisis passes, however, such doses would produce diarrhoea, as previously. Thus the body, in its wisdom, seems to be able to alter its function to meet particular requirements in this way. In order to assist a deficient immune system, such as might accompany a Candida spread, the recommended amount of vitamin C to be supplemented (in the absence of any bowel reaction) is 1–3 g daily, with food.

The effect of vitamin C on the T-cells depends of course on the T-cells being there to do their work. The thymus gland, which lies below the breastbone, can become relatively inactive, and one of the main nutrients which can enhance its production of T-cells is the amino acid arginine.[20]

A dose of 3 g daily for a short period (say a month) will boost the thymus activity at the outset of the programme, when it is most needed. *Note:* If you have a history of herpes simplex infection do *not* take arginine supplementally, for it has also been found to enhance herpes activity (this is countered by another amino acid, lysine).[21]

Take the arginine before retiring, on an empty stomach, with water. Long-term use of arginine at these levels is not suggested, although there are no known side-effects in doses lower than 20 g daily. Rough, thickened skin may develop on the elbows, for example, in doses of above 20 g daily, though this will disappear when the supplementation is stopped. The reason for suggesting a time limit to the use of arginine is that the thymus may come to depend upon such nutritional supplementation, whereas it should be encouraged to return to normal activity by the total programme of Candida suppression. Therefore take the 3 g daily for only the first month of this programme.

It is a further aid to the immune system to increase the intake of certain of the B-vitamins.[22] It is important to the programme that these are not derived from yeast sources, as anyone with a Candida problem is likely to have become yeast-sensitive.[23]

All the B-vitamins are available in synthetic forms, and these rather than yeast-derived vitamins are suggested in cases involving Candida.

Between 20 and 50 mg of vitamin B_6 (pyridoxine); between 20 and 50 mcg of vitamin B_{12}, and the same quantity of folic acid should be taken daily. Many excellent non-yeast sources of B-complex are available in the UK. (*See Further Information.*)

An additional B-vitamin (B_5) should also be taken to assist in the enhancement of the B-lymphocytes, especially if there is any evidence of allergic reactions or digestive involvement. This should be taken in the form of calcium pantothenate, at a dose of 500 mg daily. This is also useful as an aid to exhausted adrenal glands, as discussed in Chapter 4.

The minerals zinc, selenium and magnesium are all also commonly implicated in deficient immune response conditions,[24] and should ideally be added to the programme. Just as in the selection of B-vitamins, it is important to obtain a non-yeast source of selenium. Doses required of these minerals are as follows:

zinc (in the form of zinc-orotate, picolinate or citrate),
50 mg daily

selenium, 50 mcg daily

magnesium, 250–500 mg daily.

All should be taken with food.

Finally, a supply of some of the fat-soluble vitamins is called for in our effort to resuscitate the immune response. This calls for a moderate intake of vitamin E (make sure that you are buying natural vitamin E, which can be identified by the name d-alpha tocopherol, rather than dl-alpha tocopherol, which indicates a synthetic form), at a dose of between 200 and 400 iu daily; vitamin A in the form of beta-carotene, in a dose of up to 100,000 iu daily; and finally the oil of Evening Primrose (vitamin F), in a 500-mg capsule twice daily, or as one of the alternatives such as flaxseed oil.

Healing the Intestinal Mucous Membrane

If yeast overgrowth involves damage to the wall of the intestinal tract, then recolonization by friendly bacteria will be impeded. There are other dangers as well.

Writing in the *Journal of Alternative and Complementary Medicine*, Candida expert Sherridan Stock states, 'Candida damages the intestinal mucosa which leads to an increase in the permeability ('Leaky gut' syndrome) which allows large molecules of incompletely digested food protein (and yeast byproducts) to enter the bloodstream thus provoking immune responses'.[25]

There are a number of natural products which can assist in normalizing this damage. These are best used under expert guidance, however, not for reasons of risk but to ensure that what is being done is the appropriate course of action.

Among the products which may be used are:

- L-glutamine, an amino acid which enhances recovery of damaged mucous membranes

- N-Acetyl-glucosamine (NAG), an amino sugar which is a raw material for reconstruction of tissue damage and which also both assists recolonization by friendly bacteria and retards Candida's ability to 'stick' to the wall of the intestines

- Rice-bran oil (Gamma oryzenol), a superbly soothing substance which helps in tissue recovery

- Butyric acid, a normal product of the friendly bacteria, also found in olive oil, which helps in mucous membrane healing.

- F.O.S. (fructooligosaccharide) – extracted from vegetables (such as Jerusalem artichokes), F.O.S. encourages healing of the gut wall and the recolonization of friendly bacteria.

These substances may be prescribed individually or in various complexes, such as BioCare's Permatrol.

Additional assistance to the digestive process is often needed by the addition to the supplement list of enzyme complexes to assist in digestion of specific foods, and of methods for helping ensure that adequate digestive acids are present in the stomach during digestion. This might call for supplementation with hydrochloric acid capsules or more preferably with herbs which promote the natural production of acids. This will be discussed in the next chapter.

Anti-Candida and Immune Enhancement Supplement Summary

IMPORTANT NOTE

One or other of the antifungal approaches discussed above should be used, whether this involves tannates, caprylic acid and/or herbs such as berberis or echinacea, together with Aloe vera. Garlic and other substances discussed is an individual matter and normally requires expert advice.

Remember that – whatever else is done nutritionally (*see Chapter 6*) or supplementally to enhance immune function and reduce yeast-boosting foods, as well as to recolonize the digestive tract with friendly bacteria – there has to be an antifungal strategy to get rid of the yeast.

If you intend to self-medicate, then at the very least take Mycopryl 400 as well as following the immune-enhancing supplementation suggestions, the anti-Candida diet (*see Chapter 6*) and probiotic supplementation.

I urge anyone with a Candida problem to take professional advice before embarking on an antifungal programme, however, as there are so many individual variables that self-treatment can produce undue anxiety.

Lactobacillus acidophilus and *Bifidobacteria*	2 g of each, one to three times daily as recommended, in filtered or spring water at neutral temperature (Natren Superdophilus and bifidus between meals or BioCare BioAcidophilus with meals, as preferred)
Biotin (vitamin H)	350–500 mcg with acidophilus and bifidus, three times daily

Garlic	Two to three capsules daily (Kyolic brand recommended)
Aloe vera juice	Two to three teaspoons daily in water
Echinacea, hydrastis and/or berberine	Individually or in combination (as discussed earlier in this chapter)
Olive oil	Six teaspoons – at least – of Virgin cold-pressed oil daily

To enhance immune function:

Vitamin C	1 g three times daily with meals.
Arginine	3 g (with water), on an empty stomach, before retiring. Take for one month only.
Vitamin B_6 (pyridoxine)	20–50 mg daily
Vitamin B_{12}	20–50 mcg daily
Folic acid	20–50 mcg daily
	Or one vitamin B-complex capsule daily (yeast-free, slow release, high potency – containing not less than 50 mg each of the major B vitamins)
Calcium pantothenate (B_5)	500 mg daily (especially if allergy or exhaustion symptoms present)
Selenium	50 mcg daily. This antioxidant mineral is symbiotic with vitamin E and is commonly deficient
Zinc citrate	50 mg daily. Many people with candidiasis or whose immune system is under stress are zinc deficient
Magnesium	250–500 mg daily. This is commonly deficient in a Western

77

	diet, especially if immune function is under stress. This is a vital nutrient, especially indicated if fatigue and/or muscular discomfort are present
Vitamin E (d-alpha tocopherol)	200 to 400 iu daily is important for immune support and cell protection
Vitamin A (as beta-carotene)	20,000 to 100,000 iu daily. This non-toxic substance is vital for optimal immune function
Vitamin F (as oil of Evening Primrose)	One to two 500-mg capsules daily (other forms of essential fatty acids, including sources from flaxseed, borage and blackcurrant seeds, as well as fish oils, may be useful under special circumstances)

Other nutrients may also be required, including:

Chromium	(If hypoglycaemia – low blood-sugar – is a factor)
Iron	(To be supplemented only under expert guidance)
Manganese	(Important for hormonal and nerve function to be efficient)
Full-spectrum amino acids	(If protein digestion is inadequate) and individual amino acids which can only be identified by careful evaluation and testing
Nutrient combinations	Such as Permatrol (BioCare) for healing 'leaky gut' symptoms

It will be clear from the above that we are using the supplements in two directions at the same time.

First we are using probiotics and biotin (as well as herbal and other products as discussed) as substances which directly inhibit Candida and which fight its spread. The other nutrients are employed to build up the immune function (B- and T-cells) so that the body can better cope with the invading micro-organism. This part of the anti-Candida programme therefore requires that you take a large number of supplements, which can be both moderately expensive and off-putting. Let it be clear, however, that what is at stake is your health. For this reason there should be no hesitation in grasping this opportunity to fight off the cause of your ill health by whatever safe methods are at hand. The methods that are being advocated are safe. They are also effective in most cases. It can take time to control Candida once it is rampant, and six months should be seen as the minimum length of time to maintain this programme.

Yeast Die-off

IMPORTANT NOTE

During periods of rapid yeast destruction, as the supplementation and dietary programme gets underway, the body's organs of elimination (such as the liver) will be called on to detoxify the breakdown products of this process and this can lead to your feeling particularly seedy, nauseated and off-colour. The reaction is known as yeast 'die-off' or 'burn-off' and can last for some days, or even weeks. The use of proven strains of high-potency bifidobacteria, together with the general dietary strategies discussed in this and the next chapter, should minimize this. In any case do not be tempted to stop the anti-Candida programme if this process becomes evident, as this does not indicate that it is 'not working' – quite the contrary.

This is a critical stage of the treatment which, if stopped suddenly, can lead to a rebound of the Candida activity and even greater feelings of ill health. 'Burn-off' should not last for more than a week or ten days, by which time, if you stick to the guidelines given, gradual improvement should be noticed. A total control of the fungus, and therefore an eradication of symptoms, can however take many months.

Cautions and Possible Side-effects of Dietary Changes

- If you have an eating disorder, such as anorexia or bulimia, you should not attempt to change your diet radically without expert advice and supervision.

- Expect that yeast 'die-off' is a likely outcome and that this will cause odd symptoms for a week or so.

- There may be changes in bowel habits, and while these should settle down within a few weeks, get advice if there is any prolonged diarrhoea or constipation (increased water intake and linseed normally takes care of this).

- If symptoms such as palpitations, unusual fatigue, brain 'cloudiness', unusual muscle and joint discomfort, runny nose, etc. appear, suspect a food sensitivity and carefully analyse anything new in your diet, and use exclusion and rotation (as discussed for yeast in the next chapter) to identify culprit foods or substances, which should then be excluded for at least three months.

- Expect that any local yeast-affected areas will be worse for a few days. This includes oral, vaginal and skin areas. This will calm down on its own, but can be helped by use of local treatment methods as discussed below.

- If you start to crave foods (sugars and starches in particular), do not be surprised. This is commonly a result of an imbalance in blood-sugar levels due to the dietary changes, which should settle down in time. If the craving is bothersome or severe either take expert advice or use one of the following tactics.

  a Take one gram daily of the amino acid L-glutamine (away from mealtimes) and assess its effects on the craving.

  b Supplement yourself with 3 to 4 grams of full-spectrum amino acids (Lamberts' Protein Deficiency Formula is recommended) between meals, two or three times daily. This will ensure a balanced blood-sugar level.

  c Also take one Glucose Tolerance Factor tablet daily (contains chromium, which helps maintain balanced sugar levels).

  d Eat (of the appropriate foods as listed) little and often, with snacks between meals and one late at night before bedtime.

Local Vaginal Anti-Candida Treatment

There are a number of approaches which may be useful for soothing inflamed vaginal tissues during anti-Candida treatment. Whichever is used it is imperative that a comprehensive antifungal dietary approach is also followed or a recurrence of thrush or yeast-caused vaginitis will take place.

1 a Using a special soft-tipped disposable applicator, insert a solution of high-potency acidophilus culture. This can be mixed with pure water or even, more usefully, mixed with a little dilute Aloe vera juice. Any of the acidophilus

products recommended for dietary use can be employed in this way.

b   Another way of achieving this effect is to puncture an acidophilus capsule with several pin pricks and to insert the capsule deep into the vagina overnight. The acidophilus will leak out of the capsule and inhibit yeast, and the empty capsule will be expelled when douching (*see below*).

c   Mixing a teaspoonful of acidophilus powder or the contents of two capsules with live yogurt and inserting this is another means of achieving the same effect, although this will be messy.

d   Douching with water which has had acidophilus (1 teaspoonful of powder) dissolved in it will also be effective.

2   Aloe vera juice alone, diluted (two teaspoonsful in half a pint of water) can be used as a douche to relieve itching and burning.

3   A cream derived from mountain ash berries (*Sorbus aucuparia*) has been shown to have powerful antifungal and soothing properties when applied locally into or onto the vagina (marketed in the UK as Cervagyn). The active constituent, potassium sorbate, is a common food preservative (antifungal agent) but in much higher concentrations prevents yeast proliferation by interfering with its ability to feed off carbohydrates (sugars). In studies of 37 women with vulvo-vaginitis using potassium sorbate in a 1 per cent strength, there were only 11 recurrences of candidiasis over a three-month period. When a 3 per cent solution was used there were no recurrences at all out of 32 women after six months. There was also rapid symptomatic

relief where yeast was the sole infecting agent. Where other micro-organisms were involved, other methods were also needed. Results were uniformly better when the diets of the women involved were low in sugar of all sorts.

4   As mentioned earlier in this chapter, the tannate extract 'Tanafem' is available for use as a douche. This combines irreversibly with yeast cells, deactivating them and also preventing their adherence to the walls of the vagina.

5   Tea tree oil, as a pessary or used diluted in water as a douche, is an effective (if slightly irritating at first) antifungal treatment for vaginitis of yeast origin.

6   Dilute vinegar (or lemon juice) douches, on their own or with acidophilus powder added, are useful for soothing irritated vaginal tissues and for acidifying the area. Being more acidic improves the environment for friendly bacteria and makes it more difficult for yeast to adhere to the walls of the vagina. *Never* use neat vinegar on these sensitive tissues.

7   Soothing antifungal Calendula pessaries are available in Europe (including the UK) at some specialist health food outlets (such as the Nutri Centre in London – *see Further Information*)

Colonics and Enemas

Colonic irrigation involves the administration of water into the bowel, sometimes combined with other substances, in order to clear debris from the region and to encourage its health. Useful in this respect are garlic extract, oxygen and acidophilus (or as

Crook suggests, nystatin). By making repeated applications of water coupled with one of these additives there is every chance of greatly influencing the condition of the bowel. Enemas are less effective, since they penetrate only a short distance, unlike the colonic which can pass water the length of the large bowel. The technique requires expert skills, and its use in Candida problems would require additional knowledge. In principle, however, such treatment is recommended, at least in the early stages of the programme.

A caution is required as to excessive use of colonic irrigation, since this can actually deplete the normal flora if done too frequently. Its use should be limited to an actual need, precise prescription as to the number of applications and, essentially, reimplantation of friendly organisms as part of the process.

Yeast Desensitization as a Method of Controlling Candida

Carefully controlled doses of Candida extract may be injected in the hope that this will produce a response on the part of the immune system. Antibodies thus produced by white blood cells are useful in assisting the defence against antigens entering the system because of the yeast. The use of yeast extracts as a 'vaccine' of this sort also appears to assist general immune function, by helping to balance or regulate aspects of the system relating to 'helper' and 'suppressor' cells, as discussed earlier (*see Chapter 2*).

The whole exercise is complicated in the extreme, because while *Candida albicans* is a strain of yeast which is clearly identifiable, it contains within its make-up a large number of variables. Thus the Candida which is growing in one person is not exactly the same as that growing in another. This biological individuality applies to yeasts just as much as to every other living creature, including people. Thus the same extract of Candida, injected into two people, will not produce the same response. Not only is the yeast likely to prove different from that to which the individual is normally exposed, but his or her individuality, superimposed upon that fact, makes for a process of trial and error in achieving a response which is going to help the individual's immune system to fight the particular strain of Candida present in his or her system. Hereditary factors may largely be responsible for the differences in response of individuals to such treatment, and this requires that whoever is employing anti-Candida desensitization treatment be expert in the field and be able to cope with the complex variables.

Even should such expertise be available, this approach, with all its possible pitfalls in terms of variable reactions, can at best deal with just one aspect of the problem. It may assist in bolstering the immune system against the byproducts of Candida's infestation. This is especially desirable for those people who are suffering from the type of allergy symptoms mentioned earlier. But it will do little for the local symptoms currently active in the bowel or reproductive system. Only those aspects of Candida's harmful effects which are mediated by the bloodstream will be helped. Valuable as this may be, it would leave much of the underlying condition the same, and would still necessitate that the programme of anti-Candida diet and supplements be implemented, in order to control its spread and deny yeast its nutrients.

Truss points out that the use of this type of 'vaccination' programme is contra-indicated in patients suffering from what are called auto-immune conditions. These include rheumatoid arthritis. Stimulation of the immune response in someone who is being attacked by his or her own immune system would lead to aggravation of this condition. Truss has written:

I obtain yeast from supply houses that have been made aware of the necessity of bio-assaying each new batch on humans. Prior to their being informed of this fact, they were putting out a number of batches that would not give a positive skin test on known reactors. The preparation as I order it, is simply Candida albicans 1:10.[17]

This indicates one more pitfall in this method: it is vital that the Candida extract used is actually active, and that this has been proven in each batch produced, otherwise the pitfalls described above are compounded.

Our next consideration is the importance of combining the supplemental attack on Candida, and the enhancement of the immune system, with a dietary programme which deprives the yeast of its main sources of food.

Chapter 6

THE
ANTI-CANDIDA DIET

Before examining dietary strategies related to Candida problems, it is important to comment on the need for a sound environment for digestion in the stomach. Many people who suffer from 'dyspepsia' and 'heartburn' are not in fact the victims of excessive acid, but of too little, and their symptoms represent what happens when

A   their food is not adequately digested in the stomach, leading to excessive fermentation and gas, and

B   the activity of yeast in an environment which is not sufficiently acidic to inhibit them.

In 1985 researchers showed that *Candida albicans* needs a slightly alkaline environment to thrive (pH of 7.4), while in a strongly acid environment (pH of 4.5) it is completely inactivated. People taking antacid medication may therefore be encouraging yeast activity in their stomachs and digestive tracts.[1]

Dr Stephen Davies in his book *Nutritional Medicine* (Pan, 1989) lists some of the common conditions which are associated with too little hydrochloric acid, and these include: asthma, food allergy, iron and vitamin B_{12} deficiency (and therefore fatigue), bacterial and yeast bowel overgrowth, arthritic symptoms, diabetes, underactive thyroid gland, bowel sensitivity and eczema.

Among the causes of inadequate acid secretion in the stomach can be exposure to toxic pollution (such as DDT), marijuana smoking and excessive coffee consumption.

As a first step in normalizing such a problem, a strategy can be used in which hydrochloric acid capsules are taken with each meal ('Betain HCl'). If this eases symptoms significantly then a herbal method for stimulating the production of digestive acid is suggested, involving the taking of a teaspoonful of Swedish Bitters (a combination of herbs such as dandelion) two or three times daily about 20 minutes before eating.

Digestive Enzymes

A second digestive strategy may also be useful, especially if food intolerance or allergy is a feature of your condition. This calls for the supplementation of natural enzymes – chemicals which we produce to break down foods – which may be inadequately available for a variety of reasons.

A broad-spectrum enzyme combination (such as 'Digestaid' or 'Spectrazyme') is suggested for anyone with sensitivity or allergy symptoms.

If bloating and 'acid-stomach' symptoms are also a feature of an allergic condition, then Betain Hydrochloride and/or Swedish Bitters supplementation is suggested as mentioned above.

There are two primary dietary approaches which have to be considered in treating Candida overgrowth. The first involves the possibility that you may have become sensitized ('allergic') to yeast and its byproducts because of your Candida problem. As explained, this is more likely if your condition is chronic (ongoing) and if your intestinal tract has been irritated and possibly damaged by the fungal form of Candida.

If this is the case, avoidance of foods derived from yeast, or contaminated with moulds, is essential for a while. The guidelines for achieving a yeast-free diet will be explained below.

A strategy called *desensitization* uses minute dilutions of yeasts to reduce this sort of allergic reaction. This is described at the end of the previous chapter *for your information only*, as it is complicated, expensive and not always successful. It is important, however, that you are aware of this option as it has helped many people who have become 'super-allergic' and because some allergy experts might recommend the method.

Both Dr Truss and Dr Crook strongly advocate the dietary approach to treatment of Candida, especially in the prevention of Candida spreading. They are also supportive of desensitization methods.

My own view is that the dietary approach alone as set out below, combined with the anti-Candida methods described in the previous chapter, offer the best and safest way forward for anyone with a health problem caused by aggressive yeast overgrowth.

Foods Derived from or Containing Fungi and Yeast

The following list of foods and substances contain yeast or yeast-like substances, and so should be avoided as much as possible during the initial stages of dealing with Candida infection by anyone who is sensitive to them. It is probably wise to maintain vigilance about these foods for at least three months, after which time a degree of relaxation can be exercised, with the proviso that if such foods are reintroduced, and symptoms which had become quiescent begin to become active again, you should return to a stricter mode of eating for a time.

The rationale behind such avoidance is that in practice these foods seem to aggravate a Candida-induced condition, especially if allergic symptoms are part of the picture, as well as if there are symptoms such as bloating and intestinal gas.[2]

In a letter to me Dr Truss states:

If someone has no symptoms, I see no reason to have him avoid these yeast promoting foods, although I will say that in excess, and combined with a high-carbohydrate intake [sugars, etc.], these may actually induce this condition [Candida infection] even without the stimulatory effects of antibiotics, birth-control pills, cortisone, etc.

Is there any proof of the value of such restrictions?

Space does not permit discussion of all the information which proves that these restrictions are valid means of reducing the load on the immune system which repetitive allergic reactions cause, but details of one report will show their potential.

In a study of 50 patients with chronic urticaria (an allergic skin condition), all of whom had Candida antigens in their blood, it was found that more than half reacted (with acute skin eruptions) to yeast supplements and over half were said to be 'clinically cured' of their condition after following a low-yeast diet and antifungal therapy.[3]

When people are yeast sensitive/allergic it is often found that they have a reaction to a wide range of fungi, from many possible sources. It is best therefore that these are eliminated in the early stages of the programme to reduce stress on immune function.

Yeast-Promoting Foods and Substances

The following foods contain yeast as an added ingredient in their preparations,[1] and are therefore undesirable, especially in the early stages of an anti-Candida programme:

- yeast spreads (Marmite, etc.)
- breads (non-yeasted wholewheat or soda bread or corn bread is usually acceptable unless there is a grain sensitivity)
- cakes and cake mixes
- biscuits and crackers
- enriched flour
- buns, rolls and pastries
- anything fried in breadcrumbs (fish fingers, etc.).

The following contain yeast, or yeast-like substances, because of the nature of their manufacture, or of their own nature:

- mushrooms
- truffles
- soya sauce
- stock and soup cubes
- buttermilk and sour cream
- black tea
- all cheeses (especially aged or blue cheeses), including cottage cheese (some experts allow this)
- citrus drinks if canned or frozen
- all dried fruits (high mould presence on their surfaces)
- all fermented beverages, such as beer, spirits, wine, cider, ginger ale. All malted products (cereals, sweets or dairy products which have been malted)
- all foods containing monosodium glutamate (which is often a yeast derivative)

- all vinegars, whether grape, malt, cider or anything else. These are frequently used in sauces and relishes, as well as in salad dressings, sauerkraut, olives and pickled foods.

NOTE

There is disagreement among experts as to the wisdom of excluding vinegar and similar products (sauerkraut, pickles, olives) from an anti-Candida diet, and there are certainly benefits to be gained by taking apple-cider vinegar – but only if no negative reactions are observed. A simple test would be to introduce this (a teaspoon in warm water two or three times daily) and to keep a careful note of any changes in your symptoms (*see Chapter 7 for details of how to do this*).

The following are either derived from yeast or contain elements that are derived from it, and so should be avoided for at least three months of the anti-Candida regime if you show any sign of a sensitivity to yeasts or moulds:

- antibiotics
- multivitamin tablets (unless specifically stating that they are from a non-yeast source)
- B-complex vitamins (*see Chapter 5*)
- selenium (as in *Chapter 5*)
- individual B-vitamins (as in *Chapter 5*).

Dr Truss singles out some foods from this long list as the main culprits in his eyes.

He states: 'It is my belief that there are several foods that are primarily to be avoided. These include all fermented drinks, as well as vinegar, mushrooms, and mouldy cheeses. I allow my patients to have cottage cheese, as well as yogurt.'

He goes on further to say, 'It is rational to remove all of these foods from the diet, only if there is an indication that patients are having trouble with yeast Candida.'

Elimination/Rotation

If you have any doubts about whether any of these foods are likely to be a problem for you, then you should eliminate that food for at least one week and then reintroduce it twice in one day. If no reaction occurs, such as immediate palpitations, sudden fatigue, unusual brain 'cloudiness' or the return over the next 24 hours of regular symptoms which have been absent or quiescent, then you can probably include the food in your diet once more. The safest way to do this would be in a 'rotation' pattern in which you eat the food no more than once in four or five days, until the programme is well established, say after three months.

The (almost complete) elimination of all yeast-based foods, alcoholic beverages and vinegar (and its byproducts, as listed) as well as giving up blue cheeses and mushrooms, make up one part of the major dietary changes required for the first few months. The other key change involves the elimination/reduction in intake of refined carbohydrates and foods rich in sugar, which we will now consider.

Sugar-Rich Foods

Sugar (sucrose) itself, in whatever guise, is to be strictly avoided during the battle to control Candida. This means white sugar, brown sugar, black sugar and any shades in between. There is no such thing as a healthy sugar. We do not need sugar, as such, for health, and its sole claim for our attention is its taste, which it is quite easy to do without. All sugar will aid the growth and proliferation of yeast. This includes syrups, honey (yes, I'm afraid so) and other forms of sugar such as fructose, maltose, glucose, sorbitol, etc. It includes molasses, date sugar, maple sugar and in fact all of that range of non-foods with which our real foods and beverages have been sweetened. Sweets, chocolates and all soft drinks should also be totally avoided.

The inclusion of honey may come to you as a surprise. I myself had assumed that honey was relatively safe, in that it did not seem, to my knowledge, to become mouldy. I was corrected by Dr Truss, who communicated the fact that honey does indeed contain yeast spores. He pointed out that 'species of Zygosaccharomyces, a yeast, have been found particularly active in causing yeast spoilage of honey.'

It is known that honey is hygroscopic (it absorbs water) and that at a certain degree of moisture content there will be sufficient water at the surface to lower the concentration of sugars to a point that the yeasts and bacteria which might be present can grow.

Thus yeasts and other micro-organisms capable of surviving in concentrated sugar solutions (in which no yeast will grow), become able to thrive at a certain point in the dilution of that medium. In order to prevent this from happening, honey is heated and often has additives mixed with it, such as sodium benzoate, which inhibit the growth of fermenting yeasts. Truss and Crook both insist that honey be added to the list of banned foods during an anti-Candida campaign, and this is also my view. The length of time that this will be necessary will depend upon the speed of your recovery. It should not be anticipated to be less than three months, and is more likely to be six.

The undesirability of eating yeast-containing foods removes from the scene bread, pastry, biscuits and cakes, etc. This is doubly necessary since these are in the main undesirable because of their high carbohydrate content (unless totally wholegrain).

Any carbohydrate which has been refined beyond the simple grinding stage is undesirable. Wholewheat, oats as employed in making porridge, or millet, or brown rice are all highly desirable foods, rich in what are known as complex carbohydrates. These can, and indeed should (especially oats) be a part of the diet.

Once these are broken down into fine flours and are refined further they become less desirable, and actually become food for the yeast, rather than for you.

So even in the middle stages of the programme when, hopefully, your symptoms are on the wane and you might justifiably feel that you can relax the stricter aspects of the diet somewhat, please remember that refined carbohydrates are the natural food of yeast, and Candida will thank you for delivering such foods by a rapid expansion of its activity. As Truss puts it, 'Decreased availability of carbohydrates slows the rate of multiplication of yeast cells, and thus should reduce the amount of yeast products entering the bloodstream.'

The opposite is true as well: the more of these foods there are in the diet, the greater will the chances be of further spread of Candida. So out of the diet goes anything but wholemeal pasta, pastry, flour products of all sorts, biscuits, cakes, buns, rolls, bread (unless any of these are made with whole grains, and without yeast or sugar, such as soda bread).

Many foods have 'hidden sugar', in that there is sugar added in the processing or preparation. These are often foods with which sugar is not usually associated. Frozen peas, most canned foods and many packaged and processed foods all contain either refined flour products or sugar, or both. For this reason, as well as for the general undesirability of many such foods from a nutritional viewpoint, these should be avoided. Not only are you actually providing the favourite foods of the yeasts within your body when you eat sugar, you are also causing a degree of metabolic and physiological mayhem.

It should be recalled that until about 100 years ago, the average annual intake of sugar in Western countries was in the region of 20 lb per head. And this was only a part of a dietary pattern which included far more 'natural' vitamin- and mineral-rich foods than is currently the case. The present annual intake of sugar in the UK and USA is over 100 lb per head of the population. The human body is most adaptable, but it takes more than a century to get used to such a change in nutritional intake.

Organs such as the pancreas (the source of insulin and essential protein-digesting enzymes) are grossly overworked when sugar plays a large part in the diet. The pancreas, when faced with sugar, pumps out insulin. This has the job of maintaining the proper level of sugar in the bloodstream. Insulin is also released in response to stimulant drinks such as coffee and tea, which initially cause a release by the liver of stored sugar (as does stress). Thus a diet rich in sugar, and which contains the usual pattern of tea, coffee and alcohol (as well as cola drinks and chocolates, which also contain caffeine to stimulate this cycle) will produce a situation in which a major organ is grossly overworked. In this sort of pattern, the fluctuations in blood-sugar levels, boosted by dietary sugar and the sugar stored in the liver, and then depressed and controlled by the pancreatic insulin, have a profound effect upon a person's health and personality. At the same time it is noted that a sugar-rich diet makes it much less likely that an individual will eat enough foods containing vitamins and minerals to allow him or her to meet the minimum standards of nutrition. Thus other systems in the body become deficient, including the immune system. This whole process may of course take years, all the while accompanied by declining well-being and an unseen rise in Candida activity. Sugar has been well described as 'pure, white and deadly'.

It is suggested that in the first few weeks of the programme (say three weeks for safety) even fresh fruit should be avoided, because of its high content of natural fruit sugars. Even when fruit is resumed after the three-week break, it should exclude the very sweet melons and grapes, which are too high in sugar for the Candida sufferer (and often contain mould).

Milk contains its own form of sugar, and this too is thought to be undesirable throughout the programme. Pasteurized milk encourages Candida.[6] The exception to this is yogurt if it is 'natural and live', which will be clearly stated on its container. There are many 'dead' yogurts about, and a good many that have sugar added. These are quite unsuitable to the programme. Yogurt itself is helpful since it contains (when 'live') bacteria which inhibit Candida and which assist in the repopulation of the bowel flora.

Is There Any Proof that a
Low-sugar Diet Helps to Control Yeast Infection?

In one study of 100 women with Candida-induced vaginitis it was found that the levels of glucose and other sugar breakdown products excreted correlated well with the amount of dairy products, artificial sweeteners and sugars the women consumed. When they were placed on a diet which eliminated these there were 'dramatic reductions in the incidence and severity of their illness'.[7]

In another study it was shown that *Candida albicans* could not grow in human saliva until sugar (glucose) was added.[8]

Other Foods to Avoid

It is best to avoid smoked meats and fish, sausages, corned beef, hot dogs and hamburgers because of the substances added to them, some of which derive from yeasts.

Nuts, other than freshly cracked ones, should also be avoided, because of the degree of mould that these attract as they become rancid. Any foods which have been kept for a while, other than in a frozen state, are liable to be slightly mouldy, and these should be avoided too.

You now have a picture of the type of foods not to eat: mainly the yeast- and fungus-related foods, as well as the refined carbohydrates, and anything containing them.

Motivation

The degree of adherence to such a programme that is possible depends upon many factors, but none less than motivation. Just how much do you want to get better, and just how much effort are you prepared to make in that quest? It is really not up to anyone but you. Certainly the taking of the supplements, as described, will go a long way towards that end. So will avoidance of yeasts and foods derived from them. But by putting the whole programme together, including the sugar-free aspect of the diet, you really give the whole process a chance to work quickly, and well.

What you can still eat is varied and exciting. Below I have outlined a pattern of eating which is nutritious, tasty and above all 'anti-Candida'.

Once you have tried to follow this type of pattern for a while it is unlikely that you will ever want to reintroduce most of the 'undesirables', even when Candida is back under control.

Dietary Pattern

Breakfast: It has been found that a high-fibre diet is best suited to the resolution of the Candida problem. In Professor Jeffrey Bland's words, 'The diet should be higher than normal in fibre, using oat bran fibre to increase the absorptive surface of the faecal material and also hasten the elimination of metabolic by-products.'[9] Choose therefore from the following for a wholesome and non-Candida-supporting breakfast. In passing, it is suggested that you eat three meals a day, and that you should not skip a meal unless you are off-colour and really have no appetite.

Choose one or more of the following for breakfast:

1   Oatmeal porridge. Add a little cinnamon and some fresh ground cashew nuts for additional flavour. Use no sugar or honey. Make with water, not milk.

2   Mixed seed and nut breakfast (combine sunflower, pumpkin, sesame and linseed together, with oatmeal or flaked millet). These can be eaten as they are or soaked overnight in a little water to make a softer texture, or moistened with natural live yogurt. Add wheat germ and freshly milled nuts if desired.

3   Alternate days: two eggs, any style except raw.

4   Bread or toast (made without yeast or sugar) and butter.

5   Brown rice kedgeree (rice and fish).

6   Wholewheat or rice and oat pancakes (no sweetening).

7   Natural live yogurt (low-fat if possible) or 'virtually fat free' fromage frais to which is added a dessertspoonful of cold-pressed flax seed oil – blend well – and then add linseed and other seeds. This makes an energy-rich 'power breakfast' and is highly recommended (as long as you have no sensitivity to dairy products).

8   After the first three weeks or so of the programme fresh fruit can be added to the menu; for example, item 1 or 2 could be complemented by sliced banana or grated apple, or item 7 could have fresh fruit added, or fruit could be eaten as a major part of the meal, with a handful of nuts (fresh) and/or seeds (sunflower, pumpkin, etc.) Continue to avoid fruit juices, however.

9   Fish (not smoked) or meat (not cured or salted).

10 Wholewheat or whole rice flakes and yogurt (ensure no
    sugar in cereals). The use of muesli-type breakfast mixtures
    is in order if they are homemade. If shop-bought they will
    contain dried fruit and nuts of almost certain rancidity, and
    frequently sugar or honey as well. By the simple mixing of
    oat flakes, or millet flakes, with fresh nuts or seeds, as
    mentioned in item 2 above, it is possible to have a high-
    fibre, nutritious and tasty meal. If items 1 or 2 are eaten,
    then a high-fibre content will be ensured, and these are
    suggested as the most desirable. If any of the other choices
    is eaten, then add a heaped teaspoonful of linseed and bran
    (50:50), mixed together to the meal, or swallow at the end
    of the meal with a little water.

Remember to chew all food thoroughly, especially carbohydrates.
There is no way in which half-chewed carbohydrates can be
digested, since the enzymes present in saliva are essential to the
breakdown of these foods. For this reason it is undesirable to
drink with meals, as the liquid is frequently used as a moistening
agent to facilitate swallowing, which reduces efficient chewing. A
high-fibre meal is ideal for an anti-Candida programme. It also
ensures a steady release of natural sugars into the bloodstream,
rather than the rapid rise produced by most refined sugar-rich
foods. This helps to keep blood-sugar levels even, and avoids ups
and downs in available energy (and mood) which can be a major
cause of the craving for a 'quick sugar fix'.

   Drinks at breakfast time should consist of either green tea, Pau
D'Arco tea, china tea, herb tea (such as Rooibos or chamomile) –
all unsweetened – or mineral water; not fruit juices, however,
unless diluted 50:50 with water, and even then not for the first
two weeks of the programme.

   It is suggested that, in addition to other liquids, you drink not less than 1.5 and ideally up to 2.5 litres of spring or filtered water daily, mainly away from mealtimes.

Main Meals

There should be no great problem in eating quite splendid food even during the strict avoidance period of the dietary programme. One area of contention exists in the choice of animal proteins. It is important to realize that most commercial meat, poultry and eggs contain residues of antibiotics and hormonal substances which are fed to the animals in the process of rearing them for market. This means that regular eating of beef, pork or chicken, unless it comes from a source known to avoid such methods, is a potential danger to the success of the whole programme (and a health hazard at all times). Indeed it is not improbable that this very factor is a major, if as yet unrecognized, element in the whole Candida scenario. While the use of antibiotics and steroids in medication can be relatively easily remembered and identified in one's medical history, it is impossible to know just how much of these same substances are entering people on a daily basis through their food.

For this reason it is suggested that efforts be made to track down non-steroid-fed meat, poultry and eggs (and non-farmed fish), in which antibiotics have not been employed. In major cities this is probably possible. Such shops as *Wholefood* in Paddington Street, London, will guarantee supplies of meats and poultry free of all contamination. Lamb and mutton is less likely to be affected by this sort of additive, as is rabbit and any other game meat or poultry. Fish is safe, apart from other sources of pollution which do not concern Candida directly, and apart from farmed fish which may also have antibiotic contamination. For the duration of the diet, therefore, it is suggested that unless the source of fish, meat or poultry can be certainly identified as free of hormones or antibiotics, meat should be limited to game, rabbit (unless 'farmed'), mutton or lamb and fish from 'wild' sources.

Ideally, in order to maintain the high-fibre type of meal that is so desirable when Candida is active the two main meals of the day should include as wide a variety of fresh vegetables as is possible. These should be eaten both raw and cooked, and an excellent pattern to adopt is as follows. One of the main meals (say lunch) each day can be a source of protein such as fish, poultry, lamb, egg or fresh nuts, together with as large a mixed salad as your imagination can conjure and your appetite can cope with. The other main meal should also contain protein, in addition to cooked vegetables. The source of protein at each meal does not of course have to be based on animals. The combining of a cereal and a pulse (say brown rice and lentils, or millet and chick-peas) at the same meal ensures that adequate protein is available to the body.

What is essential is that adequate protein be eaten daily, whether from a 'safe' animal source or from the judicious mixing of complementary vegetable proteins. What is adequate for one person is not necessarily so for another. For example, people of East Asian origin require, for good health, less protein than people of northern European stock. The difference lies in the efficiency with which people digest and absorb what proteins they eat. Thus 50 g a day of first-class protein is adequate for an East Asian, while 75 g (or more depending upon activity, etc.) may be required by a European.[10]

Since natural live yogurt (a source of protein) is going to play a part in the diet, it is unlikely that the eating of protein at both of the main meals in addition to this is necessary. It should be possible to have, for example, a mixed salad, together with a jacket potato or savoury rice dish, and additional nuts and seeds for one meal, while having a 'safe' animal protein and a variety of cooked vegetables for the other. In any case the tastes and preferences of individuals will differ markedly, and the variations that are possible as to what to eat are so great that no more than broad guidelines can be given.

The essentials are:

- Avoid all yeast-based or yeast-containing foods (unless certain that there is no sensitivity to these).
- Avoid all sugar and refined cereal products, and foods containing them.
- Avoid all foods and drinks based upon fermentation (with the possible exception of cider vinegar as discussed above).
- Avoid meat, poultry and fish containing residues of antibiotics and steroids.
- Eat three meals daily.
- Ensure adequate protein intake.
- Ensure that a high dietary fibre content is maintained.
- Avoid fruit for the first three or four weeks of the programme.

Increasing the Variety of Foods

Once symptoms of Candida overgrowth begin to abate, usually after two months or so, and you find that you would like to increase the range of foods slightly, it is of course permissible to experiment a bit. This should not be before the end of the second month on the programme, and then only if there has been a marked improvement. If you then introduce one food which has been on the 'no-go' list, observe the consequences carefully. If these are non-existent, you might extend your experiment to another food after a week or so. If symptoms return, go back to basic avoidance, as specified above, until they calm down again. I am not saying that you *must* experiment in this way, only that if you feel constrained by the limitations imposed by the programme, then at least introduce such foods carefully, with the knowledge that they might (only might) upset things. If they do, this just means you must be patient for a little longer. There are many excellent books available which explain the principles of rotation diets which can help you to formulate a strategy for eating certain foods only periodically in a systematic way.[11] It is not suggested that the reintroduction of sugar-containing foods be started at this stage, other than in the very minimal sense – or perhaps introducing a little honey.

Other Essential Information Regarding Food

Moulds are present on most fruits and vegetables, and these should be kept well washed and eaten fresh, for obviously the longer they are kept, the more the mould development will be encouraged.

Yeasts also grow on grains of all sorts, and the fresher these are the better. A good many people with Candida problems are allergic to grains. This allergy may well diminish during the programme of Candida control, and a little experimentation is in order after two or three months if your symptoms generally have declined. A reminder is called for regarding nuts. Peanuts and pistachios, in particular, are subject to mould development (in the case of peanuts this is a highly toxic, potentially cancer-causing agent). All nuts, unless freshly opened by you, will contain some degree of mould, and certainly a degree of rancidity of the natural oils. Eat current season nuts, freshly opened by yourself, or else avoid them.

Apart from a little butter, and natural live yogurt, it is suggested that all milk products be avoided (Dr Truss does allow cottage cheese).

If you happen to go to a restaurant, or if friends invite you for a meal, then make sure that you stick to basics. Avoid sauces and gravy; avoid desserts; avoid stuffing, or any obvious undesirables, such as mushrooms. A meat, poultry or fish dish, with salad or vegetables, is the safest bet, and stick to water instead of wine.

What about sugar substitutes for those who cannot keep away from sweet things? These are open to question, as far as long-term safety is concerned, but in small amounts, for the duration of the programme (at least six months) they at least do not encourage Candida. Aspartame and saccharin fall into this category, but not fructose, corn syrup or any other sugar-rich substitute for the real thing. Fructooligosaccharide (F.O.S.) is sweet and does not encourage yeast. It can safely be added to foods for sweetness.

Remember that all commercial breakfast foods, such as corn flakes, are undesirable. They are processed, and most contain yeast and/or sugar products.

Water from the tap should be filtered before drinking if possible. There are many inexpensive water filters available that will remove a variety of organic substances which otherwise find their way into food, or directly into you. Most bottled water is acceptable, but ensure this is not carbonated if you have problems with bloating and gas. As for coffee and tea, this is a sticking point for many. They are undesirable, not only as sources of mould but because they stimulate sugar release from the liver, and consequently (a) pancreatic activity, which exhausts this vital organ further, and (b) the feeding of Candida by this sugar. There are other good reasons for not using tea, as it reduces the efficiency of both protein and iron absorption by the body; and coffee is suspected of involvement in certain forms of cancer. Herb teas are often better, and some have been found to help in the control of Candida and related problems – Rooibos, a South African tea used as a tea substitute and by allergic subjects, and taheebo or Pau D'Arco (helpful in catarrhal problems caused by Candida), etc., are worth trying.

Steaming vegetables is the best way to help to retain their vital minerals so often destroyed and lost in boiling. Dressing a salad with lemon juice, olive oil and a little natural yogurt can replace the vinegar or other dressings not compatible with the programme. As the programme produces its results and symptoms become tolerable, or disappear, so can a limited quantity of foods based on or containing mould or yeast be reintroduced. Wine, or real ale, in limited amounts, or tea, etc., may be taken occasionally. However, the need for vigilance must continue, because it is not the aim of the programme to remove Candida from the scene altogether, nor would this be possible. Even if the problem is attacked vigorously, with the use of antifungal drugs as well as the programme outlined above, the yeast will remain in the body.

The long-term answer, after initially controlling the yeast by these means, is to maintain a high level of immune function through your diet, in terms of its nutrient value, as well as by avoiding in the main those factors which you now know can reduce its optimum ability to defend you. This does not mean that the programme is a life sentence. It is hoped that after a while you will come to regard sweet tastes as unpleasant, and no longer crave or even enjoy sweet foods. It is also to be hoped that your new sense of well-being will help to motivate you towards following the pattern of eating suggested here more or less permanently, because you actually enjoy it as well as because it is good for you.

Other Factors

It is important not only to avoid foods and beverages containing fungal or yeast substances, but also to avoid inhaling these organisms or their spores. This is the reason for keeping well away from damp, dank places and for dealing with the presence of any mould and wet or dry rot that might be present in your environment. If there is any danger of damp in rooms, cupboards, cellars or lofts, do something positive about dealing with this, or, if at all possible, move to a new, dry place of residence. Your home might be making you ill. This advice is especially applicable to anyone who notices a worsening of symptoms in weather that is damp or muggy, or who is obviously affected by contact with mouldy or dank environments.

The availability of full-spectrum light is another important element which can improve your immune and general function.[12] It is known that the eyes contain photo-receptors which carry impulses directly to the pituitary gland, which lies in the head. This is the 'master gland' of the body and is vital for normal health and functioning. If the eyes are denied light (not artificial light, but the full spectrum from the sun) then demonstrable imbalances occur in the hormonal system as a direct result. Behavioural and physical symptoms can occur in consequence. The immune system is affected, and this is the reason for our interest. The advice to all who wear glasses, or who spend most of their days indoors behind glass, is that they should get outside for at least half an hour a day, with nothing between natural light and their eyes. If going out is not possible, then spend the time by an open window, without glasses or contact lenses. In a polluted city the light getting through is distorted to a degree, and so more exposure is required. This does not mean looking at the sun, even on an overcast day; just being outdoors is enough if your eyes are not shielded.

There are now available full-spectrum fluorescent lighting units. It has been found that health and productivity improve dramatically when such lighting is introduced into the workplace. As one of the additional supports for the immune system, the implementation of access to unpolluted, unfiltered, pure light is a positive step.

The immune system also benefits from adequate exercise. This means trying to apply the ideals set out in Dr Kenneth Cooper's book *The New Aerobics*.[13] At least every other day there should be a form of physical exercise sufficient to stimulate the circulation and respiration. A brisk walk of one or two miles is the safest and easiest form of exercise that can produce such results. The book mentioned should be read, and its graded advice followed. Its beauty lies in the way in which it is made applicable to anyone, at any stage of fitness or otherwise, so that the reader can gradually lift him- or herself to a level of optimum fitness in slow stages.

The avoidance of stress and anxiety is a fundamental need, as is the requirement we all have for what has been called TLC (tender loving care). These ingredients for a healthy life have been well described in many popular and readily available books. The requirement of the immune system for such inputs should encourage the study of relaxation and meditation and general stress-reducing methods. I have outlined a programme of stress-reduction in my book on the subject,[14] and this should be helpful in both assessing and dealing with those stress factors which affect life. In considering the overall importance of the immune system, it is worth commenting upon an area of medical research which tends to be ignored, because of its unpopular message. There is abundant proof that women who have relations with a large number of men are more prone to cancer of the womb than those who have relations with only one or a few partners.[15] Early sexual experience is also shown to predispose the individual towards diseases which should be prevented by an intact immune system.

HIV is more common among homosexuals who have multiple partners than among those who have steady relationships with a single partner. It would seem therefore that what is happening is that in close physical contact of a sexual nature there is a role for the immune system. It is assumed that if this is called upon to cope with antigens from a wide variety of different sources (remember that sperm is a foreign protein to the body) then it could well be a factor in depleting the immune response of an individual (along with a great number of other factors).

This viewpoint has been expressed in numerous medical journals since the AIDS epidemic began.[16] It points to a return to relative fidelity, in sexual terms, as being desirable for anyone who wishes to maintain an intact immune system. This does not mean that celibacy is called for, but that frequent changes in sexual partners are to be avoided – in both heterosexual and homosexual relationships, at the very least during the carrying out of a programme against Candida.

NOTE
It should be clear from the information provided earlier in this book that there should be no intake of antibiotics, steroids or the contraceptive pill during the course of the anti-Candida programme unless absolutely vital.

Chapter 7

PUTTING
YOUR ANTI-CANDIDA
PROGRAMME TOGETHER
– A TEN-POINT PLAN

In order to get a strong indication as to whether *Candida albicans* overgrowth is a feature of your health problems, carefully answer the questionnaire in Chapter 4.

The following suggestions do not take account of every possible variation but can be used as a guide as to what is likely to be successful in controlling Candida in most instances.

The strongest recommendation I can make is that you consult an expert in the treatment of yeast problems. Try to find a local expert who is either a naturopathic practitioner with sound qualifications, a nutritionally trained medical practitioner (such as a clinical ecologist), a homoeopath who employs nutritional methods, a well-qualified nutritionist or some other health care professional with appropriate knowledge and experience. If in doubt, ask for details of their qualifications and experience (*see also Further Information*).

If because of economic factors – or lack of such an individual in your area – you opt to try self-treatment I urge that you do not pick and choose which aspects you feel you want to try, but follow comprehensively all elements of an anti-Candida programme:

- antifungal methods
- immune support
- repopulation with probiotic organisms
- a basic anti-Candida diet
- use of additional and local treatment methods as indicated (such as healing the mucous membrane if there is a 'leaky gut').

Keeping Track of Symptoms

I suggest that you list your major symptoms on the left-hand side of a sheet of paper; underline each one and extend that line clear across the page. Then draw columns (lines down the page) which divide the page up into a series of 'boxes' into which, each day, next to each symptom you can enter a 'score' regarding its intensity over the past 24 hours. At the top of each of these columns enter the date on which you are 'scoring' your symptoms, and next to the symptom enter a 'value' – for example, if you decide that the worst your thrush irritation can ever be is equal to a score of '3' and that when there are no symptoms at all you would score a '0', you can decide for yourself what level of scoring the past day should be given.

This can be done with other symptoms such as 'indigestion', 'fatigue', 'headache', 'muscle pain' and so on.

The very bottom of the page, say the last inch or so, should be left open and into that, under the appropriate date, you can enter both a 'total symptom score' (add up all your individual scores for that day) as well as any short notes to remind you of special factors, such as 'started acidophilus', 'period started', 'started a cold', 'ran out of Mycopryl' or anything else that will jog your memory when you look back at the score-sheet, weeks or months later, as to what factors influenced the scores which you have kept. I suggest that you keep the score-sheet handy and fill it in at the same time each day, say just before your evening meal, or at bedtime.

The value of this is enormous since as you make changes in your programme you can judge their impact on your individual symptoms as well as on your 'total score'. This helps to unravel the sometimes complicated causative elements. For example, you may have five or six symptoms listed and only three of these may have changed markedly within the first few months of the programme. This tells you that the symptoms which improved probably relate directly to your Candida overgrowth while the others do not, and therefore require some other form of attention.

It is also useful to remind yourself of where you have been in terms of the intensity of symptoms as the weeks pass by. A satisfactory slow decline of scores is very gratifying (with minor ups and downs, which can occur for many reasons). It is also as well to know if scores are *not* declining, of course, at this may be an alarm signal that either the problem is not Candida related at all, or that the programme is inadequate. In either case it is better to realize this sooner rather than later.

Symptom Score Sheet
The example in the Table below shows the way in which you can keep track of symptoms and the individual aspects of the programme as they affect your health.

I suggest that you do not expect major beneficial changes before two months of the programme if the condition is severe, and that you anticipate that for a couple of weeks scores could increase during the initial stages, as 'die-off' occurs and the detoxification process begins. Since the comprehensive antifungal programme presented in this book calls for a great many changes, and since all of these are potentially stressful to some extent, as your body 'gets used' to the changes it is best to introduce them in stages, first eliminating allergens, then

symptom	date	date	date	date	date	date	date	date	date	date	
Tired	3	3	3	2	2	1	2	1	2	1	
Gas	3	3	3	2	2	2	0	1	2	1	
Head	1	1	2	1	3	2	3	1	1	1	
'Runs	1	1	3	3	1	0	1	0	2	0	
Skin-itch	1	0	0	0	3	0	1	1	1	0	
PMT	3	3	3	2	2	1	1	0	1	0	
Sore mouth	2	2	2	2	1	1	1	2	1	0	
Other	?	?	?	?	?	?	?	?	?	?	
Other	?	?	?	?	?	?	?	?	?	?	
Total	14	13	16	12	14	9	9	6	10	3	
Note	start prog-ramme				period began						

reducing and cutting out sugars, then introducing immune-enhancing nutrients and herbs, then starting the probiotic programme and the antifungal methods. All of this can take several weeks to get into place, and it is to be expected that some odd symptoms might appear during this time, especially regarding altered bowel function, abdominal 'noises' and quite probably some degree of nausea and or headaches/fatigue in excess of what you have previously noted. These changes indicate the onset of the detoxification process and should not be cause for anxiety – and certainly should not stop you from proceeding. This is where expert support and advice are most useful, especially if you are trying to introduce these changes single-handed without the emotional and practical support that is so useful during such a time of change.

Ten-point Strategy

1   If you regularly suffer from 'indigestion', dyspepsia, heartburn, 'acid stomach' – as well as bloating – consider the methods outlined in Chapter 6 regarding supplementation with Betain hydrochloride or Swedish Bitters to see whether these problems are not in fact due to inadequate acid supply.

2   If you are suffering allergic/sensitivity type symptoms, introduce a broad spectrum enzyme supplement with each main meal and assess the benefits over a period of several weeks.

3   If you are sensitive to yeast-type foods, eliminate these (as per the lists in Chapter 6) for at least two and ideally three months before attempting a challenge and possible 'rotation' use of the foods involved. If you are aware of dairy or wheat allergies, for example, eliminate these foods

altogether for the duration of the first three months of the programme, before reassessing their impact.

4   Introduce the sugar elimination aspects of the anti-Candida diet as outlined in Chapter 6.

5   Introduce immune-enhancing supplementation as outlined in Chapter 5.

6   After introducing all of the above, as appropriate to your condition, all the while assessing symptom scores as discussed at the beginning of this chapter, begin incorporating the other elements of the diet, as follows:

   A Introduce probiotic supplementation as outlined in Chapter 5.

   B Introduce antifungal strategies as outlined in Chapter 5.

   C If there are symptoms indicating bowel irritation (such as food sensitivities and/or previous diagnosis of IBS and/or mucous in the bowel movements and/or a longstanding and severe degree of yeast involvement), introduce methods to reduce bowel permeability as outlined in Chapter 5.

   D If there are local manifestations of yeast involvement, introduce local measures for mouth, vagina, etc. as discussed in Chapter 5.

7   If yeast 'die-off' is severe, there are strategies for reducing the toxic load using herbal and nutritional methods (nutrients such as molybdenum and zinc, or the amino acids L-cysteine or L-methionine and/or L-Carnitine for example) as well as herbal liver support such as silymarin (milk-thistle extract) and/or ginger.

8   Introduce detoxification methods which are not diet related
    – 'skin brushing', Epsom salts baths, various aromatherapy
    'essential oil' baths (see my book *Water Therapy* for
    information regarding these methods).
        Also consider relaxation, breathing retraining, yoga and
    other stress-reducing, immune-enhancing methods (see my
    book *Stress* for details of such methods).

9   If bowel dysbiosis (chronic bowel stasis, for example) is
    causing increased toxicity, colonic irrigation may be useful
    at this time, as may the use of 'coffee enemas'. These need
    to be individually prescribed according to need; no specific
    details are given in this text because it would be unwise for
    you to experiment with these methods on your own.

10 After two months a change in the programme may be called
    for, introducing modified antifungal strategies depending
    upon your progress to date. Changes in your diet may also
    be permissible if sensitivities are reduced.

Details of these ten points are outlined in Chapters 5 and 6;
because no two people's condition is ever the same, it is
impossible to give specific details which will suit all needs.

If your 'scores' are declining steadily (albeit with ups and
downs due to individual circumstances) there is every reason to
press on. If symptoms are not markedly improved after two
months of consistent application of the main elements of the
programme, it is time to reassess your condition and how you are
trying to deal with it. Expert advice is probably called for.

How Often Are You Likely to Need to Consult Anyone for Advice?
Certainly once at the start, and probably at six- to eight-week
intervals during the three- to six-month course of the
programme. In severe cases the programme may need to be

maintained for up to a year.

If special needs call for more frequent consultations/ treatments this should be established at the beginning of the course.

A *maintenance* programme is usually called for when Candida is under control, during which you need to maintain a low-sugar, low-fat diet, with wholesome nutritious and balanced food forming the major elements of the diet. At this time some relaxation of the restrictions is usually possible and the intake of nutrients is usually reduced to some probiotic supplementation and possibly a multivitamin/mineral nutrient support capsule/ tablet daily.

Many thousands of people have benefited from following the advice given in this book. It cannot take the place of individually prescribed methods which take account of your individual needs, but it is a useful starting point if you have found yourself unable to get help from your regular health advisers. Hopefully, as ever more GPs become aware of the value of this approach, you will find support within the National Health Service. Until then there is a need for you to take responsibility, to take action, and if possible to take advice.

The final chapter of this book examines some case histories which may be of value to you in evaluating similarities with your own condition.

Chapter 8

CASE
HISTORIES

Mrs S. M., aged 42

When she arrived for her first consultation in October 1991, this
woman was accompanied by her husband. At that time she
looked so washed-out and aged beyond her years that I took him
to be her son.

Her hair was lank, she was overweight and what I can only
describe as 'crumpled'. Her symptoms included a range of digestive complaints (intermittent diarrhoea/constipation, bloating,
dyspepsia); various PMT symptoms; extreme fatigue; skin rashes,
especially under the breasts, which had been diagnosed as yeast-
related; disturbed sleep – involving night-sweats and extreme
restlessness; depression, and of course vaginitis and thrush.
These symptoms were of about 15 years' duration, ever since she
had started bearing children (three so far). She was receiving
anti-depressant medication from her GP (and had been for over
a year) who supported her consulting me for her Candida
problems.

She expressed despair at her condition, and at the fact that
she was unable to be a 'good wife and mother', the role she had

chosen for herself. The programme I suggested was a strict application of antifungal strategies (low sugar, low fat, abundant complex carbohydrate – vegetables, whole grains) as well as a low-yeast pattern of eating (she had a history of sensitivity to yeast-based foods). I advised local application of Aloe vera juice alternating with dilute tea tree oil on the skin infection areas.

Specifically she was prescribed Natren brand Superdophilus and Bifidobacteria, with BioCare Mycopryl 680, garlic capsules (Kyolic) three times daily. A range of immune-supporting nutrients were also suggested. She kept a detailed symptom record sheet (*see Chapter 7*) and over the following six months her total score and individual symptom scores progressively declined after an initial ten days during which she stated 'I thought I was dying', so severe were her symptoms (nausea, headaches, lethargy, restlessness, flu-like aches). She had phoned me during this time of 'die-off' and I suggested that the intake of probiotics be increased temporarily (bifidobacteria helps liver decongestion) and Mycopryl cut, until severe 'die-off' symptoms lessened after a few days, at which time the programme was resumed.

By the third month, when I again saw her, she was significantly better, although there had been a period of about two weeks during the second month when her symptoms flared again for no obvious reason. She now looked years younger, had lost a stone (14 lb/6 kg) without any specific effort in that direction, and had regained some energy.

The programme was kept in place, unmodified for a further three months, by which time her symptoms were virtually absent. Her weight loss was now over two stone (28 lb/12 kg), her vitality restored, her skin clear and bowel function normal. She asked me about stopping her antidepressant medication and I suggested she talk to her GP about this. I wrote to him indicating that I believed that her depression was the result rather than the cause of her condition and that she could probably be weaned

119

off the drugs if he agreed. When I saw her for the fourth and last time at the end of the ninth month (July 1992) she had a symptom score sheet ranging between 'one' and 'zero' (it had been in the high twenties, relating to 11 symptoms, at the start – the 'one' which she was still scoring was because of a periodically furred tongue). Her weight had dropped over three stone (42 lb/18 kg) and she had successfully been taken off her anti-depressant medication. Her husband (who now looked older than her!) was delighted, as were their children, and she informed me they had told her 'They were glad to have their Mum back again.'

It was at this time that we relaxed her dietary pattern to allow a few treats of the sugary kind, and her last report, by post, a year following this indicated that all remained well.

This case illustrates the multi-symptomatic pattern many Candida sufferers endure; the possibility that anti-depressants will be prescribed for what is a symptom and not a cause; and the way in which a dedicated individual can put herself together again.

Mr F. S., aged 34

This young gay man, who had been HIV positive for some five years, arrived to see me in 1993 with a single complaint – Candida overgrowth in his mouth, so severe that the tongue and cheeks were covered in white patches. It is well known that with immune suppression comes yeast activity, and that a manifestation of oral thrush of this sort is extremely common among HIV-positive individuals and others with different immune-related illnesses. He had for the past few months started following a sound health-enhancing diet – which had previously been excessively sugar-orientated. He was, however, skipping meals from time to time due to work pressure, and on such days his energy levels were depleted dramatically.

He was troubled with intermittent diarrhoea and he was very prone to infection, with colds and chest infections almost every month, and his energy levels were lower than he felt was acceptable, making his work (in administration) an effort.

Clearly this was a condition which required careful evaluation as to how to help his immune system to function more efficiently. It is not wise to try to 'boost' the immune system where HIV is concerned, since there is evidence that aspects of the already depleted immune function are commonly overacting in an effort to maintain control of the viral infection. A 'modulation' of immune function is called for using selected nutrients and herbs, along with an aggressive attempt at restoring bowel integrity using probiotic supplementation.

His diet was tidied up somewhat (*see Chapter 6*) and a pattern of regular meals ('little and often') instituted.

A combination of supplementation with specific herbs and nutrients indicated for HIV-positive individuals, plus probiotics (including *L. bulgaricus*), herbal antifungal treatment using echinacea, Aloe vera and Tanoral mouthwash and gargle, as well as a general approach to bowel overgrowth of yeast (which must be tackled if oral thrush is to be controlled) has, over a period of 18 months, kept the yeast to only a mild degree of activity in this young man's mouth. His energy levels are increased, his ability to cope with stress is enhanced and the frequency of recurrent infections has reduced to once or twice a year – a normal level. Seven years after his initial diagnosis he continues to work and live a productive life with no health problems apart from a mild degree of yeast activity in the mouth when he is excessively stressed at work. He has joined a support group, has regular massage supplied free by a leading AIDS charity in London, practises relaxation, meditation and yoga – and safe sex.

Miss S. A. aged 39 (and Robert – aged 2 months)

This woman was in the early stages of pregnancy when I first saw her. She had a history of thrush going back many years, to her teens, when she had been prescribed antibiotics for acne. Subsequent episodes of cystitis, treated with more antibiotics, and a lengthy spell on 'the Pill' had reinforced the condition to the point where it was more or less permanent. The only variations were that from time to time it was even worse than the usual degree of irritation, discharge and itching. Medical attention produced no more than short periods of relative ease, days rather than weeks, and she had virtually abandoned discussing the problem with her GP.

She consulted me in early 1994 because of her anxiety over the potential ill-effects of yeast infection on her baby.

It is well known that during pregnancy yeast has an easier time in its activities due to hormonal changes, however there are fewer options open to treating Candida during pregnancy because of the justifiable concern for the embryo's health (*see 'Caution' in Chapter 5, page 68*). After careful evaluation of her diet it was clear that she was consuming excessive sugar-rich food, and this was modified in the process of prescribing a balanced and nutritious diet.

Supplementation with garlic and probiotics (acidophilus, bifidobacteria and bulgaricus) is perfectly safe during pregnancy and these were all suggested according to the guidelines I have explained in Chapter 5.

I also suggested local applications of yogurt into which acidophilus powder had been mixed, douching with Aloe vera in water and the use of non-drug pessaries (calendula for example).

The objective is to contain the condition until natural controls are once again able to exert themselves after pregnancy.

The tactics allowed Miss S. A. a more comfortable pregnancy and a safe delivery, after which her yeast activity declined to a level that was significantly better than had been the case before her pregnancy.

Unfortunately, within a few months of birth her baby was suffering from both cradle cap – a yeast infection of the scalp – and nappy rash, and he too was brought along for advice.

By keeping the baby dry (changing nappies more frequently than usual) as well as the frequent application of a talc which contained undecylenic acid (*see Chapter 5*) and calendula cream and/or paste made from acidophilus and yogurt, for irritated skin patches, the external manifestations of nappy rash were kept under control – while internal probiotic methods were initiated. The baby had regrettably not been able to breastfeed and so 'Life-Start' probiotic for babies was prescribed (this is a Natren product containing *Bifidobacteria infantis*) along with a low-sugar diet. It was suggested that fruit juices be provided rarely and even then only in diluted form.

Cradle cap is a scaly skin problem which affects many infants. It is a form of seborrhoeic dermatitis and often involves Candida as well – especially if the symptoms include red bumps, pimples or pustules. The various antifungal methods suggested for local application usually control this problem. Use of dilute tea tree oil as found in BioCare's 'Dermasorb' ointment, or Aloe vera juice, or acidophilus paste will all help, as long as the internal imbalances are also being dealt with (Probiotic supplementation and a low-sugar diet).

The outcome for the baby was a happy one, with all nappy rash and cradle cap clear within two months.

Mr E. M., aged 36

This young man, employed as a local government officer, consulted me in 1982 after seven years during which his health had declined dramatically. His major symptoms (and there were others) included bloating of the abdomen accompanied by nausea and flatulence, heartburn and indigestion. Constipation had become chronic. There was a tendency to light-headedness and dizziness. There were periodic attacks of shivering, followed by high temperature, which incapacitated him.

The onset of the condition, previous to which his health was unremarkable, came after an attack of gastro-enteritis while on holiday. Treatment had, naturally enough, been with a broad-spectrum antibiotic. In his own words,

> *For the 18 months following the gastro-enteritis I suffered all the symptoms daily, which were so severe it resulted in my being unable to attend work for six months continuously, and the remaining 12 months I attended only with massive support from my colleagues, who shared my workload, and understanding superiors who allowed me to go home, or rest, when the attacks were extremely severe.*

There had been a gradual improvement over the following years until some 12 months prior to my seeing him when, after an acute attack, this young man was left with all the symptoms described above. At that time he wrote, 'At present I am struggling to cope with each day as it comes, and deal with this extremely debilitating and distressing illness as best I can.'

In the intervening years between the onset of his illness and consulting me, he had been seen by numerous medical practitioners. An endoscopy (at Charing Cross Hospital) showed no disease of the bowel. He was checked for what is called a malabsorption problem, and again no abnormality was discerned. He went to the Royal Homoeopathic Hospital on two occasions, and consulted a herbalist, an osteopath and a medical specialist in allergies (a clinical ecologist). He had been placed on a rotation diet, which helped him to avoid repetitive contact with suspected food families, but which had little effect on his condition.

At the time I first saw him his diet was as follows. Breakfast: *bacon* and tomato or *sausages*. Rice cakes and *marmalade*. Decaffeinated *coffee* and *fruit juice* (not freshly made). Mid-morning he had fresh fruit. Lunch was a salad and baked potato plus *ham* or cottage cheese. The evening meal was either *chicken* or *pork* or *sausages* or fish and vegetables. He had rice cakes and a hot *milk* drink before retiring. I have italicized those aspects of his eating pattern which are contra-indicated in an anti-Candida diet (rice cakes are fine).

He appeared exhausted, but was a bright and intelligent patient who I felt would co-operate actively in any programme designed to assist his own recovery.

After tests – including cytoxic tests to elicit specific foods to which he might be reacting, as well as hair analysis (low in chromium, iron, manganese and selenium) – he was prescribed the following:

1 an anti-yeast, anti-fungus pattern of eating, low in carbohydrates.

2 supplements of vitamins A, E, B_1, B_2, B_3, B_6, calcium pantothenate (B_5), calcium, magnesium and manganese. Vitamin C was also added. The vitamin A was in emulsified form for easy absorption.

3 the pattern of eating was to include a seed and yogurt breakfast, a salad lunch and an evening meal of 'safe' protein with vegetables.

At this time the knowledge regarding biotin and acidophilus was not current, and the above programme, which the reader will recognize as a modified version of that given in earlier chapters, had a remarkable effect. Improvement began soon after the institution of the programme. Two months later biotin and acidophilus were introduced. When seen six months after the first visit, the report was of at least a 50 per cent improvement in all symptoms; there were still some days of exhaustion, but overall an upwards trend in his health was noted, after seven years of decline. Confirmation of the involvement of Candida came with an attempt early in the programme to introduce an organic iron supplement, in a liquid yeast-based form. This was met with an immediate return of constipation, which had more or less resolved itself. A check-up six months later found a continued improvement, with lapses in the diet producing confirmatory flare-ups. There is no reason to doubt that the condition will be kept under control, and that the health of this patient will continue to improve. A letter just 18 months after the start of the programme states, 'Please accept apologies for delay in contacting you. It is an indication of the progress we have made that I am well enough not to have to adhere so strictly. I am very much better overall.'

Mrs E. V., aged 50

This patient consulted me with a history of extreme itching and inflammation of the skin of the neck and scalp, of one year's duration. She had an earlier history of acne, which was treated by antibiotic therapy (unsuccessfully). She suffered from flatulence and had a history of colitis and a 'delicate' digestive system. She had consulted a herbalist, with little result, and a hypnotist who taught her relaxation and helped her to stop scratching the area. The condition remained as before. At the time of the consultation I was not yet aware of the work of Dr Truss on Candida and my approach was to use a nutrient supplementation, based on her general clinical picture, a nutritional questionnaire, a hair analysis and her current symptoms. Her dietary pattern was excellent (which, since this turned out to be a Candida problem, had probably saved her from far wider infestation).

She was placed on the following supplements, each taken orally: emulsified vitamin A, 60,000 i.u.; zinc orotate, 200 mg; calcium and magnesium orotates, 1 g each; chromium orotate 10 mg, and selenium 50 mcg; as well as oil of Evening Primrose (vitamin F), 1 g. I also suggested she take yeast tablets as a source of vitamin B. At this point she wrote to me (she lived a considerable distance from my practice) saying 'I am following your suggestions carefully, except for the brewer's yeast. Over the years I have tried a number of times to take it, but it creates gas and is most unpleasant.'

This set off alarm bells, for I had just read the first of Dr Truss' articles that week. I immediately revised the pattern of eating, which, while good under usual conditions, contained substances derived from yeast, and of course a certain amount of 'yeast food' such as honey and muesli bars. The patient cancelled her following appointment with the comment that, as her symptoms had disappeared, she felt the journey unnecessary. I quite agreed. A year later she remained symptom-free, including both skin and bowel condition.

Mrs D. B., aged 31

I was consulted by this woman, a computer-programmer, with the following list of complaints.

Eyes bloodshot and irritating, for the past nine months. Odd aches, in joints and muscles. Fingers slightly swollen. Puffiness under eyes (and sometimes above) after sleep. Ten years since the onset of this she had had cosmetic surgery and diuretics, to no avail. She had been on a macrobiotic diet as well, with no improvement.

Her periods were erratic and painful. Breasts swelled and became sensitive at this time. She felt unnaturally tired a good deal of the time.

There was a history in her family of bronchial problems and

depression, from which she too suffered.

Her current diet was:

Breakfast: shop-bought *muesli with added sugar* plus *milk* or apple juice (once a week she had eggs and *bacon* and *sausage* for breakfast)

Lunch: A cooked vegetarian savoury or *sandwiches*

Evening meal: Fish and rice, occasional meat

During the day she had the odd *sweet* and had three cups of *tea*, plus *sugar* and *biscuits.*

She had noticed a progressive inability to cope with alcohol. Her diet was reformed to remove the sugars and milk, and to increase complex carbohydrates. She was prescribed (after appropriate tests) vitamin B complex, kelp, oil of Evening Primrose, vitamin B_2, glutamic acid (an amino acid), and the minerals chromium, iron, manganese and selenium. Also prescribed were biotin and acidophilus, after meals. Within two months she reported that her period had been on time for the first time in years, there had been a less overall tendency to swell (eyes or breasts), and she was able to cope with alcohol. (It was in fact proscribed from her diet, which raises the problem of patients complying with instructions – a major headache for practitioners.) Three months later her condition was vastly improved, and her tiredness, bloodshot eyes and aching muscles and joints had all diminished to a point where they no longer bothered her. A year later she was symptom-free.

Miss G. H., aged 29

The tragic progression of ill health in this case is a clear indictment of the failure of many health professionals to recognize Candida when it is staring them in the face.

Before consulting me, the woman in question wrote to me as follows:

I have been suffering from Pelvic Inflammatory Disease (PID) for almost two years now. The problem started when I began to experience lower abdominal pain and feel generally unwell. I was, at the time, using the contraceptive IUD, which I had removed, believing this to be the cause of the pain. [Prior to this, it turned out, the young woman had been using the contraceptive pill, and had a history of recurrent thrush.] However, this [removal of the coil] had no effect and the pain became worse. Unfortunately my GP did not diagnose PID, and I therefore received no treatment in the early stages of the disease. Eventually I went to hospital, where the gynaecologist diagnosed PID through a laparoscopy. At that time there was some damage to the Fallopian tubes and adhesions in the pelvic area. I was put on to antibiotics, and for a time the condition seemed to improve. After a short time, however, I began to experience further attacks, and had to take larger doses of antibiotics regularly, and strong painkillers for much of the time. At times the pain was incredibly intense. In January 1983 I was admitted to a women's hospital in London for another laparoscopy. They found that both Fallopian tubes were blocked, and it sounded as though damage/adhesions in the pelvic area had progressed. Despite this I was told that the pain I was complaining of was psychological, and though they would be prepared to do tube reconstruction, for fertility purposes, there was nothing more they could do for me.

I visited a consultant, in Harley Street, in February 1983, who said that my symptoms and pain were classic PID, but there was nothing he could do to help ...

My menstrual cycle had now gone from four to six weeks. Apart from the pain, other symptoms were active nausea, stomach upset, dizziness, slightly raised temperature. I also became very depressed. In July 1983 I had surgery after consulting a leading gynaecologist at Hammersmith Hospital. This consisted of removal of the left Fallopian tube and reconstruction of the right; separation of adhesions to tubes, ovaries and uterus through microsurgery; presacral neurotomy (removal of nerve to uterus); steroid treatment to prevent regrowth of adhesions.

After this all was well until early November 1983, when symptoms began again. Although pain was not as severe, tests showed the infection was active again. I was put on heavy doses of antibiotics. It did not clear up, and I am now in my sixth week of antibiotics. The consultant told me that there was nothing more they can do surgically, and that I may have the condition for the rest of my life, and must learn to live with it. I have a very positive attitude towards getting better, and find it very difficult to believe that there is nothing else I can do to beat this disease, or at least fight it more effectively.

This patient's history indicated that she had commenced on this sad slide to ill health at the age of 12, when cystitis was first apparent, after which she began a 13-year history of vaginal thrush.

In late January of 1984, this patient was placed on the programme as outlined in earlier chapters: high fibre, low refined carbohydrate; no fungal foods; supplements of biotin, acidophilus, olive oil, zinc, vitamin F and garlic. Two months later she reported that she was feeling quite a lot better, apart from a couple of bad spells from which she recovered more quickly than usual.

A letter dated 10 January 1985 reads as follows:

I have been feeling considerably better. The pain problem is now limited to a few days a month (around period time). After my last laparoscopy the consultant said that it was the best result from that type of operation that he'd ever had. My remaining Fallopian tube was tested and is clear, so I am a lot happier in myself.

This is a clear and dramatic example of the tragedy that occurs when Candida becomes active in a young body, and of the effectiveness of the programme outlined in this book.

Miss S. R., aged 35

This young actress suffered from a continuous form of facial acne, which was both unsightly and a disadvantage in her work, as well as being psychologically upsetting. This condition had been present since the age of 14. Her past history was un-remarkable, apart from a highly stressed lifestyle, a surgical intervention (cryo-surgery) to deal with a cervical erosion, and a tendency not to ovulate regularly. When under stress in the past, her skin would erupt into very large pustules. By following the anti-Candida programme (as outlined in earlier chapters) her skin regained its normal health and she was ovulating regularly, after just three months. This improvement has been maintained for the past year.

Candida is possibly the least understood, most widespread cause of ill health currently in our midst. Precisely because it is known to be everywhere, it is largely ignored, and not even considered when diagnosis of conditions such as that of Miss G. H. (with PID) is sought. The cases quoted by Dr Truss, which include similar pictures to those described above, as well as individuals who were diagnosed as schizophrenic, manic depressive, and as having multiple sclerosis, deserve to be emphasized. All of these sufferers were restored to normality with the application of the sort of nutritional programme we have been considering, together with anti-yeast drug treatment.

A wider awareness of this diagnosis as a possibility would perhaps lead to a marked reduction in human suffering. Candida is not just a minor health irritant. It can destroy the physical and mental cohesion of an individual in a very short space of time. Prevention is by the same means as those described for treatment. The knowledge that we now have as to what makes Candida spread is easy to understand and easily put to practical use.

Self-help is always necessary, and until the profession of medicine becomes aware of the import of this knowledge it is vital. Past experience in this regard is not comforting. It can take 50 years, or more, for the penetration of an idea such as this to permeate the profession as a whole. Let us hope that with modern communication, and the help of the media, this will be speeded up in the case of Candida. The name of Dr C. Orion Truss, of Birmingham, Alabama, will eventually become well known throughout medicine. He is deserving of the gratitude of us all for his research into *Candida albicans* and its role as a cause of so much ill health.

REFERENCES

Chapter 1

1   *Lancet*, January 1987
2   C. Orion Truss, MD, *Journal of Orthomolecular Psychiatry* Vol.
    9, No. 4 (1980), pp. 287–301

Chapter 2

1   Roger Williams, *Biochemical Individuality* (University of Texas
    Press, 1979)
2   C. Orion Truss, MD, *Missing Diagnosis* (see Further
    Information for address)
3   Jay Stein (ed.), *Internal Medicine* (Little Brown, 1983)
4   C. Orion Truss, MD, *Journal of Orthomolecular Psychiatry* Vol.
    13, No. 2 (1984), pp. 66–93
5   Betsy Russel Manning, 'How Safe are Mercury Fillings?',
    Cancer Control Society, Los Angeles, 1984; *Health
    Consciousness*, April 1984, pp. 18–24; *Holistic Medicine* (USA),
    June–July 1984, p. 29

6   P. Thompson, 'Assessment of oral candidiasis', *British Medical Journal* 292, June 1986

7   Robert A. Da Prato MD, 'Fatty acid ion exchange complexes in treatment of Candida Albicans'. Report by Arteria Co., Concord, CA

Chapter 3

1   R. Williams and G. Deason, Proceedings of National Academy of Sciences (USA) 57 (1968), p. 1638; J. Bland (ed.), *Medical Application of Clinical Nutrition* (Keats, 1983)

2   Jeffrey Bland, Ph.D., *Nutraerobics* (Harper & Row, 1983); Dr Michael Colgan, *Your Personal Vitamin Profile* (Blond & Briggs, 1983)

3   Roger Williams, Ph.D., *Nutrition against Disease* (Bantam, 1981)

4   C. Orion Truss, MD, *Missing Diagnosis* (see Further Information for address)

Chapter 4

1   C. Orion Truss, MD, 'Restoration of Immunological Competence to Candida Albicans', *Journal of Orthomolecular Psychiatry*, Vol. 9, No. 4 (1980), pp. 287–301

2   W. Philpott and D. Kalita, *Brain Allergies* (Keats, 1980)

3   Dr W. Hemmings, *Food Antigens in the Gut* (Lancaster Press, 1980)

4   Reported in *Female Patient*, July 1987

5   The *Observer*, 1 June, 1986

6   E. Carlson, 'Enhancement by Candida of S. aureus, S. marcescens, S. faecalis in the establishment of infection', *Infection and Immunity* 39:1 (January 1983)

7   S. Stock, 'Conquering Candida', *Journal of Alternative and Complementary Medicine* (June 1993), pp. 24–26

8   L. Smith, 'Trouble in the Thyroid', *Health News and Review* 2:6 (1992); J. Trowbridge, 'An update on the yeast syndrome', *Health News and Review* 2:10 (1992)

9   E. Stretch, 'Clinical Manifestations of HIV infection in women' *Journal of Naturopathic Medicine* 3 (1) 1992, pp. 12–19

10   G. Jacobs, *Candida Albicans – a user's guide to treatment and recovery* (Optima, 1994), p. 5

Chapter 5

1   W. M. Crook, MD, *The Yeast Connection* (Professional Books, 1988)

2   *American Journal of Obstetrics and Gynecology* 15, 1986

3   K. Shehani and A. Ayeno, 'Role of dietary lactobacilli in gastrointestinal microecology', *American Journal of Clinical Nutrition* Vol. 33 (Nov. 1980), pp. 2448–57; M. Speck, 'Contributions of micro-organisms to foods and nutrition', *Nutrition News* Vol. 38, No. 4 (1975), p. 13; G. Reddy *et al.*, 'Natural Antibiotic activity of *Lactobacillus acidophilus* and *bulgaricus*', *Cultured Dairy Products Journal* Vol. 18, No. 2 (1983), p. 15

4   K. Shehani, 'Nutritional and Therapeutic aspects of cultured dairy products', Proc. XIX *International Dairy Congress*, Vol. 1e, 1974

5   Jeffrey Bland, Ph.D., 'Candida Albicans: An Alternative Therapy for an Unexpected Problem', *Journal of Alternative Medicine* (July 1983), pp. 18–19

6   J. Rasic, *Bifidobacteria and their Role* (Basel: Birkhauser Verlag, 1983); C. Fernandes *et al.*, 'Therapeutic role of dietary lactobacilli', *FEMS Microbiology Reviews* 46 (1987), pp.

343–356; T. Kageyama *et al.*, 'The effect of bifidobacterium administration in patients with leukemia', *Bifidobacteria Microflora* 3 (1984), pp. 29–33; S. E. Gilliland *et al.*, 'Beneficial interrelationships between certain microorganisms and humans', *Journal of Food Protection* 42 (1979), pp. 164–167

7   *Medical Science Proceedings* (Yamaguchi, 1982)

8   Jeffrey Bland, Ph.D., *Journal of Alternative Medicine*, June 1985

9   *Applied Microbiology*, June 1969; L. Harris, *The Book of Garlic* (Aris Books, 1979)

10   *Medical Journal of Australia* Vol. 1, No. 60 (1982)

11   Tyarcke and Gos, 'Inhibitory Action of Garlic on Growth and Respiration of Micro-organisms' (1979)

12   *Mycologia* Vol. LXVII, No. 4 (1975)

13   *Mycologia* Vol. LXIX, No. 4 (1977)

14   Bland, 'Candida Albicans'

15   I. Neuhauser, *Arch. Int. Med.* 93, pp. 53–60

16   Gill Jacobs, *Candida Albicans – a user's guide to treatment and recovery* (Optima, 1994), p. 237

17   C. Orion Truss, MD, *Missing Diagnosis* (see Further Information for address); Crook, *The Yeast Connection*

18   Jeffrey Bland, Ph.D., *Nutraerobics* (Harper & Row, 1983); Dr Michael Colgan, *Your Personal Vitamin Profile* (Blond & Briggs, 1983)

19   Robert Cathcart, MD, 'Vitamin C-Titrating to Bowel Tolerance', *Medical Hypothesis* 7 (1981), pp. 1359–76

20   *American Journal of Clinical Nutrition* Vol. 37, No. 5 (1983), pp. 786

21   *Dermatologia* No. 156 (1978), pp. 257–67

22   Bland, *Nutraerobics*

23   Truss, *Missing Diagnosis*; Crook, *The Yeast Connection*

24   J. Bland (ed.), *Medical Application of Clinical Nutrition* (Keats, 1983); Bland, *Nutraerobics*; W. Philpott and D. Kalita, *Brain Allergies* (Keats, 1980)

25 S. Stock, 'Conquering Candida', *Alternative and Complementary Medicine*, June 1993, p. 25

Chapter 6

1 G. Bodey and V. Fainstein (eds), 'Candidiasis in the gastrointestinal Tract', in *Candidiasis* (New York: Raven Press, 1985)

2 C. Orion Truss, MD, *Missing Diagnosis* (see Further Information for address); Crook, *The Yeast Connection*

3 Report on study by I. Holti, in M. Werbach 'Nutritional Influences on illness' (supplement; Tarzana, CA: Third Line Press, 1991), p. S13

4 Brown and Binkley, *Yeast: A Brief Description of Common Sources* (1980)

5 Personal communication to author, 1983

6 W. M. Crook, MD, *The Yeast Connection* (Professional Books, 1988)

7 B. Horowitz *et al.*, 'Sugar chromatography studies in recurrent Candida vulvovaginitis' *Journal of Reproductive Medicine* 29 (7), 1984, pp. 441–43

8 L. Samarayanake *et al.*, 'Proteolytic potential of candida albicans in human saliva supplemented by glucose' *Journal of Med Microbiology* 17 (1), 1984, pp. 13–22

9 Jeffrey Bland, Ph.D., 'Candida Albicans: An Alternative Therapy for an Unexpected Problem', *Journal of Alternative Medicine* (July 1983), pp. 18–19

10 J. Bland (ed.), *Medical Application of Clinical Nutrition* (Keats, 1983)

11 Robert Forman, Ph.D., *How to Control Your Allergies* (Larchmont Books, 1979)

12 John Ott, *Light Radiation and You* (Devin Adair, 1982)

13 Kenneth Cooper, *The New Aerobics* (Bantam, 1977)

14 Leon Chaitow, *Stress* (Thorsons Health Series, 1984)
15 Bland, *Clinical Nutrition*
16 Editorial, *New England Journal of Medicine* Dec. 10, 1981; Editorial, *Lancet* 12 Dec. 1981
17 Personal communication to author, 1984

FURTHER
INFORMATION

Supplement Suppliers

Alwyn Company, Inc.
P.O. Box 940
Mankato, MN 56002-0940
Tel: 800-793-2666; fax: 800-336-9007
Website: www.alwyn.com/myconil.html

Manufacturer of Myconcil, a wash that inhibits the growth and reproduction of Candida albicans.

Archangel Health Store
Website: www.aomega.com/ahs/candida.htm

Offers on-line purchase of all-natural health products with a full line related to Candida albicans.

Elixa, Ltd.
805 Kriss NE
Albuquerque, NM 87112
Tel: 800-766-4544; fax: 505-293-4648
Website: www.elixa.com

Supplier of Dr. Wolfe's Homeopathic, mercury-free dental products and colloidal silver generators.

Essentially Yours
Website: www.wwns.com/sanders/eyi/0-prod.htm

Producer of Agrisept, a natural, nontoxic product used as a preventive treatment that kills fungus.

Freeda Vitamins
36 East 41st St.
New York, NY 10017
Tel: 212-685-4980
Website: www.freedavitamins.com

Source of yeast-free supplements, caprystatin, and Vital Dophilus.

Great Earth Mail Order
Tel: 888-878-3842
Website: www.sweetvia.com/dooriy.html

Supplier of Sweetvia, a natural sweetener safe for yeast intolerance.

Higher Ideals, Inc.
2300 N. Main St.
North Logan, UT 84341
Website: www.mbay.net/~rhess/aqua.html

Source of Aqua Pure, a homeopathic remedy for Candida albicans.

Life Plus
P.O. Box 3749
Batesville, AR 72503
Tel: 800-572-8446
Website: www.lifeplusvitamins.com

Supplier of Ecology Pak, a nutritional program to fight yeast and establish healthy bowel ecology; MSM Plus, a biological sulfur supplement critical to healthy metabolism; and Paratox, an herbal blend specifically formulated to help the body cleanse and detoxify itself.

Natracare, LLC
191 University Blvd., Suite 294
Denver, CO 80206
Tel: 303-320-1510; fax: 303-320-3901
Website: www.indra.com/natracare/

Provider of a full line of non-chlorine bleached, natural feminine hygiene products.

Natren, Inc.
3105 Willow Lane
Westlake Village, CA 91361
Tel: 800-992-3323
Website: www.natren.com

Source of Megadophilus.

Upward Quest Health
P.O. Box 1378
Grand Lake, CO 80447
Tel: 970-627-9255
Website: ww2.upwardquest.com/UpwardQuest/Menu.html

Supplier of Nature's Biotics, a powerful probiotic.

Whole Health Discount Center
112 Havenwood Dr.
Cranberry Twp., PA 16066
Tel: 800-382-1936
Website: health-pages.com/ec/index.html

Source of echinacea, a broad-spectrum immune system stimulant helpful in the treatment of chronic, recurring vaginal yeast infections.

Support Groups

Candida Albicans Discussion
Website: www.i-depth.com/P/y/yr02016.frm.candida.html

Dedicated to keeping Candida albicans under control with natural supplements. Features a message board, chat room, and cookbook.

Candida Yeast Infections/The Yeast-Free Page
Website: www.nidlink.com/~mastent/yeastfr.html

A website featuring recipes and a newsletter focusing on mastering food allergies.

Directory

Amalgamlinks
Website: vest.gu.se/~bosse/Mercury/Mouth/Linklists/dds.html

Lists dentists who use mercury-free methods and provides facts about amalgam/mercury.

Broadway Dental Center
310 Harvard Ave. East
Seattle, WA 98102
Tel: 206-324-1100; fax: 206-324-6711
Website: www.nwdentist.com/html/home_buck___rubin__d.d.s.html

Provider of mercury-free, biocompatible dentistry.

Candida E-Mail Directory
Website: alces.med.umn.edu/candida/email.html

List of e-mail addresses for Candida albicans researchers.

Candidanews Communications
Website: alces.med.umn.edu/candida/cnews/cnews-com.html

Lists significant postings from "Candida News," a forum for the exchange of information on Candida research.

Dr. Paul Gilbert
123 Dunhams Corner Rd.
East Brunswick, NJ 08816
Tel: 908-254-7946
Website: www.holisticliving.org/Dentists.html

Provider of mercury-free, biocompatible dentistry.

Great Earth Vitamins
205 East Swedesford Rd.
Wayne, PA 19087
Tel: 800-473-2810; fax: 610-687-1180

Franco Prezia, nutritionist and herbologist, specializes in nutritional counseling for Candida sufferers. Phone consultations are free.

INDEX

BOOKS OF RELATED INTEREST

Lupus
Alternative Therapies That Work
by Sharon Moore

Healing Lyme Disease Coinfections
Complementary and Holistic Treatments
for Bartonella and Mycoplasma
by Stephen Harrod Buhner

The Transformational Power of Fasting
The Way to Spiritual, Physical, and Emotional Rejuvenation
by Stephen Harrod Buhner

The Acid–Alkaline Diet for Optimum Health
Restore Your Health by Creating pH Balance in Your Diet
by Christopher Vasey, N.D.

Optimal Detox
How to Cleanse Your Body of Colloidal and Crystalline Toxins
by Christopher Vasey, N.D.

Food Allergies and Food Intolerance
The Complete Guide to Their Identification and Treatment
by Jonathan Brostoff, M.D., and Linda Gamlin

Optimal Digestive Health: A Complete Guide
Edited by Trent W. Nichols, M.D.,
and Nancy Faass, MSW, MPH

Primal Body, Primal Mind
Beyond the Paleo Diet for Total Health and a Longer Life
by Nora T. Gedgaudas, CNS, CNT

Inner Traditions • Bear & Company
P.O. Box 388
Rochester, VT 05767
1-800-246-8648
www.InnerTraditions.com

Or contact your local bookseller